MULTIPLE
SCLEROSIS

Mission remission

Healing MS against all odds

Steven G. Fox, Ph.D.

Multiple Sclerosis Mission Remission:

Healing MS Against All Odds

Bookbaby

Pennsauken, NJ

ISBN: 978-1719442657

This is my personal story and sojourn to health by sending multiple sclerosis (MS) into remission with the help of the universe and God. It is my second book. My First book, *Dreams: Guide to the Soul*, focused exclusively on dreams. *Multiple Sclerosis Mission Remission* includes dreams as one of many important tools involved in my healing. My personal psychology enters the picture a lot, and the treatments I discuss are what worked for me. Others may not respond similarly. In my case, years of physical abuse laid the foundation for developing the chronic illness of multiple sclerosis, which is my opinion that informs this book's premise and the treatments I have pursued.

Table of Contents

Chapter 1

The Thunderclap

My vision went double. My speech slurred. I dropped things. I sometimes fell down for no reason. My wife, being the board-certified psychiatrist that she is, insisted that I consult with a neurologist. The neurologist performed numerous tests and procedures. It was time for us to meet the good doctor and hear the results.

When we went to obtain the results, the neurologist mumbled a few words and looked down at the floor while he spoke. I processed nothing of what he was saying to me. Repression is a remarkable phenomenon. He talked to my wife for what seemed like a long time. Driving back from the doctor's office to the Arizona State University Student Health Center, where my wife was the psychiatrist on the eating disorders team, Debby was uncharacteristically quiet. When we drove into Student Health and I stopped the car to let her out, I found out why.

"Well, I guess we will keep trying to figure out what is going on with me," I said with resignation.

"What are you talking about? The MS looks severe," she said. Deborah never suffered a fool well.

"MS?"

With disbelief Dr. Deborah Brogan said, "Didn't he tell you that you have MS, multiple sclerosis?"

"What?" I asked.

Debby answered, "You heard me. The doctor said you have multiple sclerosis."

So, it began, my fifteen-year journey through purgatory. I thought I must have made serious mistakes in a previous life. At the time, it seemed as good an explanation as any for why I contracted multiple sclerosis, MS. It turns out that I probably contracted multiple sclerosis because of conditions I endured in this lifetime, including the cold climate I was born into in the Midwest, abuse I had endured as a child, drinking too much diet soda with aspartame, frequent bronchitis, genetics, a car accident when I was thirty-one years old, working out in a hot karate studio, etc.

MS is a syndrome that I believe is ignited by a host of various factors coming together. I believe it to be the exception, rather than the rule, for multiple sclerosis to occur from only one causative factor. I think that is why MS must be fought on numerous fronts—it probably was caused by the totality of a life assaulted on many fronts, just as it affects every aspect of life.

At the time, I thought I just wanted to return to my old self, the "I" my ego thought of as me. I never accepted the MS as the real me, but as an adversary sent to test the real me. Little did I know how much my real self was going to change because of the battle—no, the war—against multiple sclerosis. Sometimes I think life bakes us in a mold during the first eighteen years of life, and then we spend the rest of our lives trying to break out of that mold. I used to think that happened only emotionally. I now think it happens physically as well. College and graduate school transformed my mind as an adult. MS transformed my body, mind, and spirit. The only difference among these three realms is that the spiritual changes never stop unless we close ourselves off to our humanity. In an unexpected turn of events, I had never lost so much. Regaining health seemed like it would take a miracle. After fifteen years, the miracle happened. I was previously agnostic about the possibility of miracles. I am now a connoisseur and student of miracles. I have realized that miracles are mostly finding ways out of difficulties when it seems like there is no way out. This is not Pollyannaish denial. The first step to a miracle is realizing you are in a situation where answers are not easy.

When you have a major illness, it is not the time, in my humble opinion, to hedge your bets. You start out realizing that, at least initially, you have lost the bet. You thought you had been so healthy most of your life—surely you would not contract a neurodegenerative disease. The hard truth is that when a major illness comes, a personal disaster has happened. The odds of overcoming it are slim, but you have little chance of turning the situation around until you realize how dire the situation truly is. If you want to overcome a major devastating disease for which there is no known cure, I believe your odds vastly improve if you are willing to do anything that does not cause permanent damage to fight it.

You must at least try low-probability treatments, as long as they do no permanent damage, because in many cases, it is not known what will be curative for you. I believe you have to try a no-harm, or low-risk, treatment, because for you it might be the best way to beat the thief in the night of chronic illness. The reader is cautioned that I use the words "cure" and "sending into remission" for chronic, incurable illness for one reason—when the chronic disease is sent into remission, it feels and generally looks like a cure, but do not be fooled. *After sending the disease into remission, the sufferer must still make every medical, personal, and habitual choice for health to keep the dreaded disease in remission—it is likely still lurking beneath the surface.*

You will explore the edges of the known. The internet is your ally and friend. I particularly like the Braintalkcommunities.org Neurological Disorders and Injury discussion boards. The specific board or forum regarding multiple sclerosis is at:

http://www.braintalkcommunities.org/forumdisplay.php/81-Multiple-Sclerosis

You will get many ideas from boards like these. Almost nothing works for everyone; almost everything discussed worked for someone. You must find out if that medication, treatment, energy method, diet, exercise, or lifestyle change works for you and is important to your recovery. Make sure it is a low-risk—or at least potentially high-benefit compared to the risk—treatment. You want to gather as much information from medical or other professional sources as is available.

Doctors are willing to do experimental procedures if you indicate that you are fully informed. Additionally, with my doctors, I always assured them that they did not have to worry about a malpractice suit. *Any treatment that doctors pursued on my behalf in good faith and with my full consent would never be pursued in court by me, especially when I knew there was a good chance the treatment would not work.*

My general rule for myself was that I would consider anything that had a 5% chance of helping and did no permanent damage. I was willing to accept temporary pain and inconvenience if the procedure would ultimately help me and would do no permanent damage. Your willingness to accept risk and endure pain or inconvenience will determine what personal rule will work for you. I actively dreaded the idea that I ever would stop trying to improve my disability.

Accepting MS is not a clarion call to send up the white flag and go to sleep. Accepting multiple sclerosis means realizing what a physically and mentally burdensome situation you are in. It's like getting a flat tire on the interstate in the middle of a desert. You can bemoan the fact that you have a flat tire, but whining will do you no good and get you nowhere. Getting out of the car, getting outside of yourself, and figuring out what spare tire or parts you can find to fix the situation means accepting that you have a flat tire and must find help and make a change.

Information is vital. Communication is paramount. It is important to set up a communication system. In the case of the flat tire, you want a smartphone to get information, such as how far it is to the nearest gas station. You obviously need a phone to call for help. With MS, you similarly need every device and avenue available to gather information. The computer can be particularly helpful. You want information from the internet, books, and experts so you can obtain the best medical and alternative care, and can adopt the best personal practices (diet, exercise, sleep schedule, daily routine, recreation, and so forth).

I was in a state of shock, and I was surprised that the medical doctor talked to my wife about my condition instead of to me. My wife was a physician and a board-certified psychiatrist. The doctor, I supposed, thought it was easier to tell my wife first. I now believe that he did tell me, but I did not want to hear any of it, so I repressed what he said. Being a psychologist does not guarantee that my mind will not defend itself with bold-faced repression. The subconscious is always measuring how much information we are ready to accept.

His gut instinct was to make this a doctor-to-doctor consultation first. It was my hypothesis that he did not want to endure another patient's reaction to a conundrum in life. I thought his instincts were good. The truth was my subconscious did not allow me to process the horrible news until I heard it from someone I loved: my wife.

I was a licensed psychologist in private practice, and I was thirty-six years old at the time. Ironically, even though I was married to a psychiatrist who regularly and almost always prescribed medication to her private practice patients, I was largely unenthusiastic about the use of medication. I preferred to minimize the effects of biology on development, considering environmental influences equally or more important.

I saw psychotropic medication as an adjunct to psychotherapy in most cases of anxiety and depression. Anxious and depressed clients made up the bulk of my private practice. I knew that medication could be helpful in many cases.

I thought medication was most helpful in cases of extreme anxiety, major depression, and psychosis, and especially attention deficit disorder. There were some cases where medication was almost mandatory, such as bipolar disorder and schizophrenia. I did not know it at the time, but the first part of my bio-psycho-social view of people was going to be emphasized. I was going to be given a lesson in biology I would never forget.

I frequently tell people that, in my limited experience, medication tends to positively improve a patient's major depression or psychosis on average from 20% to 40%. With attention deficit hyperactivity disorder (ADHD), if the right ADHD medication is used for a specific person at the correct dosage, the improvement in symptoms tends to be at least 40%, and I have seen as much as an 80% improvement. There are cognitive and behavioral interventions that help, but to get the fastest relief from symptoms, it's usually best to start out with medication and then use behavioral/cognitive methods to ignite further positive changes. As with Maslow's psychological theory of self-actualization, basic needs must be met first before addressing needs more aligned with the higher self.

As will be seen throughout this book, I have shifted toward the belief that a bio-psycho-medical-behavioral-alternative-spiritual approach stands the best chance of producing miracles. In my view, we must deal with basic biological and medical needs first. Once that building block is in place, more progress can then be made in the other spheres. One can use, and I believe it is important to use, intuitive alternative spiritual/psychological approaches to help decide what interventions are most likely to work for a given person. It is not body versus mind, but body *and* mind, strengthened through biological, intuitive, alternative, and spiritual approaches. You must find what works for you. In the process, you find out more about who you really are. It seems as if the universe often makes the most of this devastating event to force us to change—it may not be what we personally planned. The main choice we have is how we are going to react to this horrific event.

Biological views of myself were literally going to be emphasized on steroids. The major biological intervention against the degenerative multiple sclerosis (MS) would be a combination of steroids with other medicine. But I am getting ahead of myself. First, let me elaborate on why I wrote this book, and explain what I think multiple sclerosis is.

Chapter 2

Why Did I Write This Book?

This is my story about having multiple sclerosis (MS) for fifteen years before all the various treatments reached a critical mass and sent it into remission. The book's structure alternates between portions of my personal story and chapters that describe a treatment method. Rather than follow a rigid structure, I present the admixture of treatment methods with my personal story according to what feels natural or necessary. For example, the initial chapters, mostly about diagnosis, are followed by a chapter on visualization, which is vital to many, if not all, of the alternative methods employed.

I describe the medical treatments by necessity; they are central and core to my personal story. Pharmaceuticals plus alternative treatments worked together to produce the MS remission. It is never a question of Eastern versus Western treatments. I believe the solution to sending chronic disease into remission is almost always using Western medicine combined with Eastern alternative methods. We do not want to be biased according to what we wish were true. We want to throw everything we possibly can at the disease, with the order of interventions following this general rule: **Western methods are usually best for an initial acute injury, followed by Eastern alternative methods, which are usually most helpful when applied to chronic conditions that have no known cure.**

I think Western medicine is best for acute traumatic injuries, infections, and recently contracted diseases. Once the initial treatment has been followed medically by Western methods, I believe Eastern treatments can offer more in many chronic situations. The East has millennia of experience dealing with chronic illness without the benefit of our modern-day offerings of Western medical care. The East developed its own methods, independent of Western medicine, that can be used to further a patient's long-term recovery. Once Western medical treatments have stabilized the situation, Eastern alternative methods are best at preventing the injury or disease from getting worse.

Eastern exercise, such as yoga, and an Eastern or a Mediterranean diet, are often considered beneficial for prevention. One could discuss at length the massive relaxing and healing effects of energy methods such as Reiki or hot stones on your chakra points while Reiki is being performed. These positive effects are not meaningless fluff, but techniques for mastering the body's long-term ability to heal once the body has had sufficient time to heal, rather than being assassinated by the initial insult/attack/episode of disease.

The essential point is that this is not a competition between mainstream and alternative methods. Each has value in a comprehensive treatment plan. We can learn from stories like that of Steve Jobs, the founder of computer giant, Apple.

Steve Jobs died relatively early because he thought he would try more natural methods rather than starting out with mainstream medical treatment. Right before he died, he stated that he would have had a better chance of survival if he had sought standard medical treatment earlier. **In the short-term initial stage, the West is best. When the illness becomes a chronic beast, go East.**

By the time you know you have a major illness, such as multiple sclerosis (MS), you are so far behind the disease that it is necessary to use whatever treatment works for your individual situation. Eastern and Western approaches are complementary.

Which treatments will work for a given individual? The only way to find out is to obtain the best expert advice you can and try various methods until you determine whether the method or medicine is likely to be helpful. This book details the different methods that worked for me.

Will they work for you? It is likely that not all of them will work for you. It is also likely that some of them will work for you.

Each person has a different biological structure. It is unlikely that everything that worked for me will work for you. It is also the case that at least some of the methods I used are likely to work for you. We are each unique, but we are all humans.

You must be willing to actively seek treatments that may work for you. Moses was lost in the desert for forty years trying to find the promised land. Consider this book as a road sign to get you to healing faster. It may be no coincidence that I'm writing this book from the middle of a desert, in Phoenix, Arizona.

Some methods, such as psychotherapy and dreams, primarily help with discernment. Dreams and therapy helped me to decide what treatments to pursue. Dream incubation, described in my first book, *Dreams: Guide to the Soul* at www.drstevenfox.com, is a way of specifically asking your subconscious personal questions and then receiving answers in dreams.

Dreams are usually right 90% of the time unless the dreamer is seriously mentally ill. My conscious self tends to be right about 70% of the time on a good day. I would rather be right more often.

It is true that the conscious mind can be insistent, even when wrong. We often consciously think what we want to hear, which may not be true. The subconscious can be uncanny about being right because it usually tells us what we need to do, not necessarily what we want to hear.

This is a quest. It is the quest of your life. This journey ultimately can give your life a new perspective. Life and illness asks a question—how are you going to answer? You can give up, lie down, and die, or you can fight. If you are brave enough to fight, I can guarantee you only one thing. **It will be the fight of your life.**

This book describes remission from multiple sclerosis because that's the chronic disease with which I was dealing. I believe many of the methods described will work for people with other chronic diseases as well. We are all biological beings. In my view, we have energetic and spiritual realms that are greatly affected by our cognitive and subconscious processes. Many of the methods described will probably work with many people because these techniques are good for health, mind, and spirit—that is my hope, wish, dream, and prayer for you.

You may be thinking: just exactly what is multiple sclerosis, anyway? Let us now delve into the anatomy of this complicated neurological disorder.

Chapter 3

What Is MS?

Multiple sclerosis is an autoimmune disease in which the immune system mistakenly attacks the nervous system. Specifically, MS targets the fatty myelin covering nerve fibers in the brain and body. Myelin speeds the nervous system impulses so that your movements, reflexes, and thinking are much faster. Myelin amps your internal computer (your brain) and the cables (nerve fibers) that lead to it. Myelin, metaphorically, is insulation over electrical cords. The myelin protects the nerve impulses and allows the electrochemical impulses to travel much faster. This insulation makes quicker and more complicated processing possible in the brain and nervous system.

Myelination is the process through which more and more of the nervous system, including the brain and the spinal cord, is covered by the impulse-speeding myelin. Myelination has profound effects upon a person's development. It turbocharges the nervous system. It is more than a quantitative improvement. It is a qualitative leap that allows theoretical and hypothetical thinking that could not have been previously processed.

At the age of thirteen or so, the brain goes through a major increase of myelinated nerve fibers and brain neurons. The speeding of brain pulses allows for complex thinking. It turns the elementary brain into a supercomputer now able to deal with abstract concepts. This growth spurt in myelination is most noticeable in the adolescent's newfound ability to do algebra problems and talk for hours about God, the meaning of life, and political concepts. The person now has the tools to define a self-identity.

The brain continues myelination well into the early twenties. This may explain why, if one begins chronic marijuana use before the age of eighteen, it can have harmful effects on cognitive functions. Intellectual abilities were reduced in adolescents who used marijuana heavily over an extended period. The decrease in intellectual functioning was not found in persons who started using marijuana after the age of eighteen (Meier, Caspi, Amber, et al., 2012). The adult brain is further developed and more capable of withstanding assaults. A completed fortress withstands attacks better than a fortress with defenses still under construction when the attack begins.

Thus, MS is a many-not-so-splendored thing. Its symptoms depend upon which part of the nervous system the immune system is attacking. Vision is usually affected first, followed by balance and coordination. It can affect hearing and speech. I personally found the slurring or change in my speech to be the most distressing. It can affect sensitivity of touch by producing feelings of numbness.

It mercifully seems to affect the higher levels of abstract thinking the least. It does not appear to significantly reduce life span. On the other hand, people afflicted with MS are not likely to live to be one hundred years old. MS has made me a much stronger believer in the importance of quality of life. I would rather have eighty years of relatively good-quality life than a hundred years of less-than-mediocre life.

Were there any early warning signs of multiple sclerosis (MS) symptoms for me? Scanning my life for predictors of MS, I remember my vision blurring unexpectedly several times per day when I was twenty-eight for about two months. I started checking my vision several times per day by focusing my sight on the tip of a finger. It randomly became blurry at times. I could occasionally detect some minor double vision. It disappeared after those two months, not to return until I was thirty-six years old. This was a warning and an omen. Multiple sclerosis often presents first with changes and damage to the optic nerve.

Let us now look at something that can be useful for everyone with a chronic disease—visualization.

Chapter 4

Visualization

The main concept holding most of the various alternative methods together is visualization. It is hard to overestimate the value of visualization. I believe that if you visualize something, your subconscious, at some level, acts as though what you visualized has happened. If you fantasize about something, there is the potential that the subconscious will use that fantasy as a blueprint for action when the opportunity presents itself.

This is not to say that we can do without physical processes. Visualization works best when anchored by the body. For example, weights and exercise work better if the person visualizes how they affect the body while doing the exercise. It is important for the body to respond to the feedback it gets from the brain. It is equally vital that the mind focuses on the commands it is sending to the body. Visualization and focus constitute the mustard seed that moves the mountain of chronic illness. The kingdom of God is within. The human mind is very powerful.

Stem cell biologist Bruce Lipton, in his book *The Biology of Belief*, presents a strong argument that thoughts can influence which DNA cells are activated to use protein to repair the part of the body focused upon. DNA is a system that can be profoundly affected by your thoughts. When fighting a chronic illness, you are in the business of cell repair and re-repair. Visualization helps the brain more directly connect with the body to conduct restorative processes.

Let us talk about basic strategies to employ conscious visualization. Before performing the exercise, you need to watch your trainer, yoga teacher, physical therapist, or god/goddess (who is preferably some combination of these) do the exercise. You need to meditate on it and visualize it to the point that when you start to do the exercise, it feels almost like a repetition, because you are only now physically doing what you previously mentally ingrained into your subconscious. With determination and spirit, you convince yourself that you are going to do this despite whatever obstacles stand in your way. You are sending an unfiltered message from your mind to your brain, your body, and the universe that you are a force that flows with and into healing.

With practice, you come to feel that you are the exercise. The exercise is playing you more than you are doing the exercise. Through repetition and devotion, with solemn dedication that is uninterested in excuses, you become the exercise, and this helps your body find new pathways to travel to your muscles. The body is replete with replication. I believe that frequently the damage is not directly repaired so much as the mind/body finds new ways to get the nervous signals where they need to go. New pathways are created.

There are many far-flung methods I will describe that have this core foundation—visualization. If you deeply visualize a repair to your body and believe it, your subconscious will assume that what you have visualized has happened to the degree that you really believe it. If you only believe it a little, that is how much it will help—a little. A strong belief that you are having a positive effect upon your health will overcome many barriers. The subconscious responds to repetition. Your body will believe you are healing to the degree that you practice belief in healing commands. You only must be willing to try to believe.

There is no placebo effect. There is mostly the effect of what you believe. If you believe that a pill (which in someone else's eyes is fake) will work, it will have some effect. Not necessarily because of the pill, but because your belief has mobilized the power of visualization. Your belief has added to the power of the pill, or the belief by itself can cause positive effects. Is it the medicine or your belief that heals? The only proper answer is yes. The only sure thing in my world is that dedicated and applied belief will almost certainly have a positive effect. The pill may or may not have the desired effect—that is best left to science. Healing is best left to the person it matters the most to—you.

I want to convey the process of how I did this. It may work for you, but you must have discernment, which you can improve with many of the methods that follow. In other words, you can use some of the treatments, like psychotherapy and dreams, to help pick out the means that are likely to work for you. Our subconscious knows us best.

Dreams are where the subconscious talks directly to us. We need to listen, particularly when we are wrong. We want to take things based on trying and then feeling or discerning whether there is movement toward health from that effort.

I want to emphasize that I believe the processes I used will work, with modifications, for many people. These methods are likely to be helpful for other major diseases as well. The medicines will be different, but the alternative treatments will likely be similar because most of these methods are ancient, field-tested over millennia, and have been found to be beneficial to humans.

These therapies are often ancient, but frequently reimagined with a new twist. That new twist may be the modification a certain segment of people need to turn the corner on a disease. People are different and yet similar. We all share different modifications of the same biological structure. Consider the analogy of a car: while there are many different types of cars, most can be driven using the same basic driving skills, with some modifications.

The application of the alternative methods to specific conditions is where the rubber meets the road and discernment is necessary, especially where prevention of future attacks is paramount. I want to give examples of how my visualization specifics are dependent upon my background. We want to pick visualizations congruent with our unique selves, including our upbringing, and our current beliefs. We want to grease the wheels of healing by initially going with whatever positive spiritual and therapeutic beliefs you already have.

By picking things congruent with our upbringing, we elect to swim with the river instead of swimming against it. There is a wealth of childhood images that have the advantage of already being installed and entrenched in your personal subconscious. In this case, we do not have to work on ingraining these images in the subconscious because they are already there. We can use these ingrained beliefs as a starting point to build upon other related positive beliefs.

Our ingrained beliefs from most major religions and philosophies are mostly positive. While avoiding the controversial or negative parts of those beliefs, we can build upon a base of universally accepted tenets. Negativity is not allowed. You cannot afford it. No one with a chronic illness can afford to lease part of the mind out to negative beliefs. Pessimism is a virulent part of any chronic disease. The antidote is usually hope.

The clearest examples I can give of something that worked for me involves my Catholic upbringing. These images may not work as well for someone else, unless they truly and currently trust in them. The Catholic Church is expert in instilling certain images in children's minds. The Church frequently has believers in its hold from birth onward. It takes more work to eradicate brainwashing that took place from birth to adolescence from the mind than it does to just accept the parts of the faith that work for an individual as an adult and disregard the rest.

In fact, the Vatican is so expert that even if, later in life, a Catholic decides not to believe everything the Church teaches, there will often be emotional uneasiness around the ingrained subconscious thought that maybe, just maybe, there was some truth in what they taught you—and there's the rub. There undoubtedly was some truth in what they taught you. The fallen-away Catholic many times returns to the fold later in life, often probably to hedge their bets. Sometimes bucking the system can cost the sufferer more energy than the patient can afford to expend.

I went through Catholic elementary and middle school. All religions vary in how well the brainwashing is instilled. Religions do not equally instill their own unforgettable images and beliefs in children. To be maximally effective, the images and beliefs are presented dogmatically with no room for error. The Catholic Church is good at this dogmatism. Its leader, the Pope, is considered infallible in matters of religious doctrine.

Fortunately, we know from history that the Church is anything but infallible. The Church's insistence that the Earth was the center of the universe did not make it so. Some of these beliefs were undoubtedly self-serving, but they also may have been held for the benefit of humanity given the period back then. If you are living in squalor in the Dark Ages, it might have been some consolation to believe that God placed you at the center of the universe. It would give you some basis to believe that maybe humankind was important.

I have taken the path of accepting Catholicism, but with a more expanded view of the universe. It is my proclivity to honor all religions if the thoughts mostly go up and not down. This is the basic position of an omnist—believing that all major religions have some positive contribution to make. It is a compromise I can live with.

I believe this is a compromise that the world should eventually make in order for all of us to share earth peacefully. My beliefs eventually bent this way because of the necessity, as a psychologist, to be able to work with many different people of many different faiths. I now accept the major tenets of most major religions for two reasons:

1. The central tenets of the major religions converge toward truth, and

2.   These central tenets tend to be the same, or highly similar.

For example, I like the tenets of Buddhism. I could convert to Buddhism easily, apart from my realization that I would feel mostly like a Catholic imitating Buddhists because of my subconscious images. It is, frankly, easier to add the philosophy of Buddhism to Catholic leanings than to accomplish the reverse feat. Buddhism seems to have few, if any, negative beliefs. It is a philosophy that fits nicely and synergistically with other worldviews.

It seems to me more productive to build upon what I know and transform that material like clay on a potter's wheel. Destroying what you know and building belief anew with unfamiliar concepts is fraught with difficulty. You are left with an inner child who has nagging questions about what religious leaders instilled in your brain, namely, *I wonder if they were right?*

All of this is my way of saying you must find the images that work for you. I devote chapters to angels and saints because that is what worked for me—it also just plain feels good to me. More importantly, it feels reassuring. This is important because the subconscious is conservative in protecting you. Above all, the subconscious is strongly biased against making any decision that could endanger your being. I believe working with the subconscious makes healing more likely. Different religions, different philosophies, and unique individuals each have their own stellar, memorable images. I prefer more positive viewpoints. For example, Reiki (which will be described extensively in later chapters) seems to be nothing but positive, with no downside, which is why I incorporate it into my more universal outlook.

This is not to say that strong beliefs we have acquired on our own can't have an equally strong transfixing effect. New beliefs can sometimes have an even stronger hypnotic effect on the fervent believer. A good example is my acquired belief in Reiki following my experience with Reiki masters.

Visualization of your personal, strong images is, I believe, the most likely of the alternative methods to help turn the tide against the villain from hell called MS. You really do have to see it within your mind to convince yourself that something the so-called experts say is highly unlikely, such as complete remission from multiple sclerosis—the big MS—is possible. ***If you have this disease or another major illness and you somehow do not think you are in a major cosmic battle, you are missing the point. You are in the battle—no, the war—of your life.***

Follow your subconscious to the internal visualization of what you want, and not what this demonic illness has planned for you. You do not have to be religious for this to work, but being spiritual does help. At the very least, you must believe in yourself.

You need undivided focus. If you have an attention deficit, it needs to be treated. Medication for attention deficit is the most successful psychiatric medication there is, in my experience, given what patients have reported to me after being treated by their medical doctor.

Depression and anxiety reduce attention. If you are depressed, you need to be treated. Comorbid disorders lessen the chance for success. You need all the energy you have to counter the illness. You must get rid of any other energy-sapping conditions you have.

I have always operated from the principle that if you are building a house and it is on fire, you need to put out the fire first. That is why the emphasis is initially on doing the acute medical care. When your body is on fire with an inflammatory disease like MS, Western medical care is the nearest fire extinguisher. Eastern beliefs and treatments seem better in maintaining the temple of your body after it has been rebuilt.

Depression is also inflammatory, and you almost certainly will be depressed. We even talk about the "kindling effect" of depression. That is, once the cycle of major depression starts, it has a reinforcing, cyclic effect—you become more depressed with the realization that you are depressed. Also, once you have major depression, there is increased risk later in life that you could relapse into depression. That is the bad news.

The good news is that most people with major depression will recover repeatedly. That is, most depression is relapsing-remitting. Most multiple sclerosis is thought to be relapsing-remitting in the beginning. It was thought that my MS was relapsing-remitting for the first five years I had it, but it was not.

After four or five years of slow gradual decline, it was thought that I might have secondary progressive multiple sclerosis, but I did not. After descending further into increasingly severe symptoms, it was finally realized by the brilliant neurologist Timothy Vollmer, who was with the Barrow Neurological Institute, that the correct diagnosis was the granddaddy of them all—primary progressive multiple sclerosis.

Since it is likely you will be experiencing some degree of depression with MS, it is important to get this inflammatory condition—depression—under control. Medication and psychotherapy is what worked best for me. Fortunately, most antidepressants also have the secondary effect of lowering anxiety. You must be of sound mind to beat the formidable foe of chronic disease. Psychotherapy helps you make the best health-creating decisions.

You also must be willing to admit to yourself that no one knows with certainty what can and cannot be accomplished with the help of belief. If we believe the words of avatars like Jesus Christ, it is a lot more than what a person with a major illness can imagine. And besides, you have nothing to lose but your disbelief. You might regain most of what the illness took.

In any case, this process of self-discovery while recovering from a major illness is beyond any drug-induced state. LSD will show you pretty pictures but will not get you to where you need to go, and may do harm along the way. You cannot afford any more damage when you are fighting a chronic illness. You will rediscover the natural high of being who you were meant to be.

Chapter 5

The Breakdown

In my thirties, I started learning karate. I initially studied Okinawan or Japanese karate before moving from Albany, New York, to Tempe, Arizona. Tempe is next to Phoenix, and is the home of the massive 80,000-student and growing Arizona State University, where my wife was employed as a psychiatrist. Right before the MS was detected, I was in Taekwondo.

Karate is a Japanese martial art that emphasizes the hands and the punch. Taekwondo is a Korean martial art that emphasizes the legs and the kick. I wanted to learn the discipline of self-defense and to present a more confident persona. Little did I know that these Eastern arts would be instrumental in detecting the MS.

It is probably more accurate to say that the martial arts triggered or unmasked the underlying multiple sclerosis. Heat can unmask multiple sclerosis. Sometimes the heat source can be something as trivial as a hot shower. I guess there was always a reason I was leery of saunas. In my mind, water was meant to cool one down.

I was in the Taekwondo studio at the age of thirty-six, getting ready for testing to be promoted from a red belt to a brown belt. Things really start to rock and roll as a red belt—you do things like crack a concrete building block. Looking back on that, I can hardly believe I broke a building block in two. Being accepted into the brown belt was preparation for the ultimate black belt. It was a life goal, but time ran out.

The studio was very hot in the days prior to the brown belt test. The head, or sensei, of the studio liked to let the temperature go over ninety degrees in sunny Phoenix, Arizona. I was practicing my routine, and the black belts noticed that my kicks were not as sharp as usual. My coordination was poor, which was never a problem for me previously. I fell doing an easy high kick, and the studio suddenly became silent and still. A black belt tried to ask me what was wrong. I did not know what to say.

I picked myself up and left, thinking I must be getting too old for the tricks. I was embarrassed to the point that I gathered my things and fled. I knew something major was wrong. Little did I know I would never return.

Not becoming a black belt would later become a loss I would grieve for the person I never became. It's funny how physical achievements rank high on the list of things we are likely to remember as we age. I guess I realized how vital the physical realm was to life when I could no longer physically do what I once could.

I retreated to my private psychologist practice office, which then was in Tempe, Arizona, in the East Valley next to Phoenix. The office was only a stone's throw away from Arizona State University (ASU). My wife was on staff at the ASU Student Health Center as a psychiatrist and was on the eating disorders team. It often felt like Arizona State University was the de facto eating disorders capital. ASU was one of the largest, if not the largest, universities at the time, and has grown impressively since then.

It was disconcerting that when I went to a nearby bistro, I frequently and spontaneously dropped my oversized Pepsi Big Gulp container for no reason. I was not indoctrinated in the evils of soda at that time. I often wonder if drinking nearly a six-pack of diet soda per day for three years at my first job in Albany, New York, contributed to my getting multiple sclerosis. Aspartame, the diet soda sugar replacement, has been shown to be neurotoxic. I saw diet soda as probably egging the MS on. It probably was more of an aggravator than a causative factor in my multiple sclerosis.

Nowadays, water is my preferred drink. It is naturally refreshing, and it is free. It's funny how it usually costs more to buy things that hurt our health. Worse than that—we later must spend more money to try to regain health, which may or may not work. An ounce of prevention truly is worth a pound of cure. That is because it is much easier to stay healthy when we are healthy than it is to try to restore ourselves to a previously healthy state.

Let's see: so far, I had past vision problems, reduced strength, dizziness, and poor coordination. I was literally "losing my grip." I thought that surely things would not get worse. They did. I did not realize it would involve my speech.

The topper, and the symptom that finally drove me to the neurologist's office, was that my speech became slurred. This was at the height of the initial MS attack. Slurring my speech as a psychotherapist was horrific. I stopped the practice and headed for the doctor as fast as I could. My speech had never been great, but this symptom announced to the world there was something desperately wrong with me. At that point, multiple sclerosis was literally "in my face." No pun intended.

The first neurologist I saw defined his role in my dilemma as a diagnostician. He first did a CAT scan. A CAT scan is often the first step to try to get some idea of what is going on. CAT stands for Computer Assisted Tomography. Two-dimensional image slices of the brain are obtained to rule out tumors, strokes, or head trauma. My CAT scan indicated further investigation was necessary. When you are told that further tests are necessary, it's often the prelude to an "oh no" moment.

The neurologist then did a spinal tap, which was not so painful, but felt as though something was leaving my body that should have been left alone. I lay on my side on a cot while he stuck a needle in my spine to withdraw the spinal fluid. This procedure rules out serious infection in the nervous system. No infection was found. I expected this result.

The final procedure was the decisive Magnetic Resonance Imaging (MRI). I was placed horizontally, head first, into a metal tube. It takes between ninety minutes and two hours; the range depends upon whether images of both the brain and spinal cord are requested. It usually is a good idea to do both, because multiple sclerosis virtually always eventually attacks the spinal cord. The procedure also takes longer if they ask for images with and without contrast. In that case, you receive a transfusion of dye halfway through to light up the images and make them clearer.

Powerful magnetic waves produce three-dimensional-like images to see if there are any lesions. An MRI is not unpleasant unless you have claustrophobia and cannot stand enclosed spaces. They give you earplugs because the machine makes a lot of noise, including clicks and what sounds like someone is banging on pipes with a pipe wrench. Multiple sclerosis (MS) causes white lesions to appear on the MRI images.

The whiter the image, the more demyelination has taken place. My MRI images lit up the screen like a search light—there was so much white that one should have worn sunglasses. There were massive lesions in my brain, and some lesions in my spinal cord.

This was not a case where your future is so bright, you gotta wear shades. I have always had a sort of gallows humor about disease that I suppose helps me to cope with my chronic illness. In many ways, I think having a sense of humor about the situation implies a certain acceptance of the situation.

What did the bright white on the MRI mean? It meant I had MS, without a doubt. The neurologist gave me 60 mg of Prednisone daily to stop the attack, which it did. Prednisone also gave me racing thoughts and the feeling that I was ready to jump out of my skin.

Because my father had bipolar disorder, or manic-depression, since his forties, I believe the doctors decided that giving me racing thoughts was not a good idea. It is interesting that when they later gave me intravenous transfusions of steroids, my thoughts sped up, but were far from racing. The delivery of the steroids was crucial for me.

Whether it goes through the stomach as a pill or is delivered directly intravenously by an infusion makes a big difference in how the medication affects me. In my case, I virtually always prefer an infusion to a pill. The processing that is performed on the medicine before it is delivered to the body is, I believe, a major complication that may be related to the many side effects we see with pills.

I bet the same pills have different effects on many people because of differences in digestive systems. When using a pill, you put a major intervening variable—your digestive system—in the way of a cure. Prednisone would be the first of many pharmaceutical interventions in this tale of continually trying something different until a therapeutic effect begins.

Chapter 6

Good Luck Strikes and the Standard Treatment

Shortly after I was diagnosed, the first medicine to prevent MS attacks successfully, Betaseron, was approved in 1991 by the FDA. I thought it was synchrony, or a meaningful coincidence, that I started to show severe MS symptoms at about the same time Betaseron was developed. I think its major contribution may have been that it showed MS could be treated. For me, Betaseron probably prevented further severe acute MS attacks from recurring, but it lost some of its effectiveness after I used it for many years.

They held a lottery to determine which patients would receive the Betaseron medication first because there was a shortage. Good luck struck. I was one of the first patients in Arizona to receive Betaseron. It was the first and only lottery I have ever won. I thought maybe my luck was changing.

My neurologist will go unnamed, simply because he meant well. He was old-school, as he was well over fifty years old. Before the 1990s, there was not much a neurologist could do in the way of treatment for multiple sclerosis. When he went through medical training, neurologists were like pathologists. They mostly could correctly diagnose why you were going downhill, but could do little about it. Neurologists were seen almost strictly as diagnosticians. Being a neurologist then meant being fascinated with ascertaining the presence of mostly hopeless diagnoses. He was well-schooled.

The situation had changed with Betaseron's introduction. It was a change in basic assumptions about MS. This then-new medication, the first of its kind, mostly prevented MS attacks for people with relapsing-remitting multiple sclerosis. Hallelujah!

Relapsing-remitting MS was diagnosed when the symptoms varied from severe symptoms at times followed by periods of remission, that is, a lessening or disappearance of symptoms. I was diagnosed as having relapsing-remitting because they did not really know initially what kind of multiple sclerosis I had. Also, they wanted to try Betaseron on me, which was effective for both relapsing-remitting and secondary progressive MS. It was the go-to medication of the time.

The long-range view regarding the overall picture was that once you had MS, it would stay that way forever or get worse. That certainly was the prognosis if you were diagnosed with primary progressive multiple sclerosis. It was later determined, from the course of my illness, that I had had primary progressive MS from the start.

I had a hunch maybe a person could send MS into permanent or semi-permanent remission simply because I noticed that my symptoms changed from day to day, often depending upon how well I was taking care of myself. I saw, even after being diagnosed with primary progressive MS, that I could have a positive effect on the course of the illness by following beneficial health practices.

From that standpoint, there was good news and bad news. The good news was MS symptoms tended to change, often a lot—for good or ill. The bad news was that the long-term trend in the changes was that symptoms tended to get worse or spread to new areas. In any case, the disease tended to have periods of at least temporary, even if minor, improvement. Being a *Mission Impossible* fan, I saw my mission as permanent remission—*Multiple Sclerosis Mission Remission.*

I planned to make a dent in the hopeless scenario envisioned by well-meaning, but frustrated, healers or those simply wearing white coats with no healing to offer. I resolved that I would do anything that was legal or moral that had a 5% chance or more of improving the MS symptoms. I did not think there was one silver-bullet treatment that worked for all comers.

Multiple sclerosis is a many-legged monster that needs an army of healers to defeat it. In fact, defeating it requires more than just an army. You also need the air force, navy, national guard, green beret, marines, navy seals, homeland security, FBI, CIA, NSA, mercenaries, drones, outer space surveillance, and the joint chiefs of staff. Add to that a lot of meditation, prayer, synchronicity, and luck. You are long past the point of having the luxury of taking your time to decide which treatment may comport with your worldview.

You need to use anything morally acceptable that may help move the needle toward a cure. You must be willing to learn to accept more help than you ever knew existed. You negotiate, if you will, at the United Nations for peace while preparing troops for attack. Meditation, relaxation, and prayer are your allies. You ask any credible spiritual or religious group to pray for you.

I believe that the person with MS must do numerous interventions, until the patient reaches a critical mass, or tipping point, that propels the patient into remission. I think it was synchronicity (a meaningful coincidence of unrelated things that seem related because of the way they occur) that this new medication came to market shortly after I developed MS. At the time, I thought Betaseron significantly lowered the chance of future MS attacks, and, subjectively, it seemed to improve my symptoms. If I liken improving my health to building a house, it is important to first put out any house fires before continuing to build the house. Betaseron looked, at the time, to be one of the first fire extinguishers.

Betaseron did not make anyone MS-proof or fireproof. Its main contribution was that it gave more time for additional fire departments (other treatments) to arrive. It seemed to work for me at first, before complications set in. But I am getting ahead of myself again.

My first neurologist and I tried various approaches. Once we even tried an anti-rejection drug, Imuran, also called Azathioprine. This drug, for people with transplants, keeps the immune system from attacking and rejecting the newly transplanted donor organ. At the time, it was used mainly with kidney and heart transplants. Kidney transplants at that time were almost 90% successful. Less common transplants, like liver and pancreas transplants, were much less successful. Stronger and different anti-rejection drugs were needed for different organs.

Logically, it should have worked. Tragically, it did not work. Biological systems are often more complex than man's reasoning. We often do not know exactly why something works or does not work. The human body is a complex thing that can either heal itself or attack itself.

My neurologist had spent years in frustrated failure treating MS. His first instinct was to throw cold water on ideas hopeful of sending multiple sclerosis into complete remission. He did not know that I was married to a woman who was predicted to die before she was in her forties because of severe juvenile diabetes.

She became a doctor, received a kidney-pancreas transplant, and worked until she was almost sixty. All this despite being legally blind from her twenties on due to the severity of the diabetes. He could not imagine the example of determination to stand up to chronic disease that my wife had given me.

My first neurologist tried to console me, mainly by assuring me that the situation was hopeless. He would look at my worsening symptoms and sometimes drift into the philosophical realm. He once remarked how little effect medications in the past had in improving the condition of the MS patient despite initial enthusiasm. He had a sort of learned helplessness that was irritating at best and infuriating at worst. In a way, he helped me develop an intolerance for those insisting that acceptance of the disease meant being okay with the idea that there was little to do except wait to die.

He was not going to become slap-happy and agape at the historic success of Betaseron. While gazing in the distance, he opined, "You know, multiple sclerosis symptoms tend to wax and wane." I guessed he considered MS variation as certain as the changing of the seasons. It seemed very biblical in the sense "to everything there is a season." Fortunately, in that biblical passage, there is no reference to "a time to have MS." The passage (Ecclesiastes 3:1-8) is as follows:

1. To every thing there is a season, and a time to every purpose under the heaven:

2. A time to be born, and a time to die; a time to plant, and a time to pluck up that which is planted;

3. A time to kill, and a time to heal; a time to break down, and a time to build up;

4. A time to weep, and a time to laugh; a time to mourn, and a time to dance;

5. A time to cast away stones, and a time to gather stones together; a time to embrace, and a time to refrain from embracing;

6. A time to get, and a time to lose; a time to keep, and a time to cast away;

7. A time to rend, and a time to sew; a time to keep silence, and a time to speak;

8. A time to love, and a time to hate; a time of war, and a time of peace

The person fighting MS will experience all of these times. Let me draw your attention to verse 3. There is indeed "A time to kill, and a time to heal; a time to break down, and a time to build up."

When you acquire multiple sclerosis, you have experienced a time to break down, and you, of course, need to rebuild. Paradoxically, your time to heal will probably occur when you decide, with the love of God inside you, to kill the MS. It needs to be a righteous killing of a disease that has taken much from you and wants to take all. You will feel the force of healing and gain energy from the spirit of the universe flowing through your body if you are able to channel it right.

Most of my first neurologist's verbalizations seemed to be, on the positive side, to tone down my enthusiasm for new treatments to spare my mental health from disappointments. On the other hand, taking such a stance probably reduces the risk of malpractice suits because of patient disillusionment with new treatments. Doctors may sometimes be reluctant to share optimism because they instinctively want to avoid inflating a patient's expectations. God forbid patients have too much hope!

It seems more nefarious to err on the side of giving no hope whatsoever. It is, however, far easier to defend in a court of law. Patients and society pay an enormous price for malpractice suits.

There were other drugs introduced during my slow slide into noticeable symptoms from 1997 until 2005 in addition to Betaseron. They included Avonex, Copaxone, and Rebif. They came to be known as the ABC-R multiple sclerosis drugs. They were all for the relapsing-remitting type of multiple sclerosis. I had different reactions to the drugs, none of them absolutely positive, because I was later correctly diagnosed as having primary progressive multiple sclerosis, which may not respond to the relapsing-remitting MS drugs.

Avonex was a once weekly, deep intramuscular, self-administered injection. I thought it genuinely helped. The main advantage of Avonex was that you did not have to think about the MS as much. To have three or four less times per week that you did not have to think about multiple sclerosis, by giving yourself an injection, was heaven. The change in self-concept that MS imposes is a burden.

Betaseron was an every-other-day, self-administered injection that, until complications close to the end of my Betaseron usage, seemed to help. Betaseron was always the old favorite, and I returned to it several times. I usually gave myself the every-other-day Betaseron injection in the upper part of my thighs. Sometimes I gave myself the injection in the fat of the abdomen, which I initially thought would hurt unbearably, but it did not. I guess my expectation of inordinate pain from the abdomen shots came from childhood memories of watching television shows where rabies victims were given dreadfully painful abdomen shots.

Betaseron had the disturbing habit, every so often, of killing skin near the injection site, which left a small scar. I still have an assortment of these small scars which, fortunately, if I keep working out, blend in with my minor six-pack. Betaseron was also indicated for secondary progressive MS—which I was optimistically diagnosed with because of my long, slow slide into more severe symptoms.

The overall course of events proved that I had the worst form of MS, primary progressive. I gradually developed incontinence, worsening balance, and increasingly poor gait. My heat sensitivity became more severe. I was headed toward a wheelchair, the horror of horrors for a previous long-distance runner.

I tried Copaxone at one point. It was a daily and relatively minor subcutaneous injection. I have no positive or negative feelings about Copaxone. It seemed to neither help nor harm. It simply did nothing for me. The daily reminder that I had MS was annoying. Giving myself a daily injection that did nothing to improve my condition did not help my morale.

The European contender for treating relapsing-remitting multiple sclerosis by preventing MS attacks and flare-ups was Rebif. It was worse than nothing for me. In my world, it would have been better called Regress because it genuinely seemed to make my symptoms worse. One wants to keep in mind the warning Hippocrates, often called the Father of Medicine, gave: "First, do no harm" when considering a treatment. My dizziness, numbness, poor coordination, weakness, and fatigue raged on with the so-called treatment of Rebif. Doctor recommended or not, I decided to reject Rebif before it killed me.

My first neurologist asked at one point, when we seemed to be running out of options, "What would you be willing to do to get rid of MS?"

My reply was out of my mouth almost before he finished his question: "Anything."

He remarked, "I was afraid you were going to say that."

When doctors know they have a patient willing to take risks, they feel they are taking risks with their career. Most innovative treatments involve a certain amount of risk because they are new and have not been validated by thousands of people. You must convince your doctor to take risks for the following reasons:

1. You have nothing to lose.

2. He will be blazing a new trail.

3. You are fully informed and agree to take all risks.

4. Most importantly, if a doctor performs a procedure in good faith that you consented to with full knowledge that you could die, neither you nor your estate would ever sue.

He was afraid of doing harm, while I was mainly afraid of not getting better. I did not want to outlive my health and be trapped in an unresponsive body. I had tried all the ABC-R drugs, which were Avonex, Betaseron, Copaxone, and Rebif. I was ready for a new drug and hoped it would overinflate my wildest hopes.

I will later talk about Tysabri, which turned out to be the miracle MS-attack-prevention drug that also seemed to improve my symptoms.

I can write in cursive much better now at age 64 than I could when I was 40 years old. The more I use Tysabri, the better I get. It is so successful, in my case, I am afraid of outliving my money.

With Tysabri, there is some danger that you could get a rare brain virus; however, there is a test they can perform to determine if the virus is latent in your brain. It is called the JC virus.

If you do not have the virus, there is little danger of complications, to my knowledge, but you need to check with your doctor who knows your medical status. For example, Tysabri is probably not a good idea if you have an active infection. It is significant that I am more prone to get colds when I am taking Tysabri, which is why I avoid shaking hands. Knowing what I know about disease and immune systems now, I cannot understand why many medical doctors insist on shaking patients' hands. One of the most effective means to avoid spreading disease is to wash your hands.

I do want to mention that there is a new MS medication, Tecfidera, that prevents MS attacks. The advantage of Tecfidera is that it is a pill, and you do not have to deal with those god-forsaken injections. I have not taken Tecfidera, because Tysabri fulfilled my MS medication needs. I also was not interested in Tecfidera because it is a pill that my digestive system would be likely to affect.

I have decided to stick with Tysabri since it is an infusion I do only every six or seven weeks. I recently was in danger of becoming JC virus positive, so I lengthened the interval between infusions to reduce risk. The infusion does not involve the hassle of injections and has had no side effects for me, which I cannot say for many of the other medications. Tysabri has done more than prevent my symptoms. In combination with the other exercise, diet, and Eastern methods I use, I think Tysabri has repaired, replaced, or modified nervous system pathways so that I continue to improve on a neurological basis.

Five or six years after my diagnosis, around 1998, my falls were becoming a weekly event. I once fell outside when leaving a doctor's office and separated my shoulder, and experienced profuse bleeding from hitting the back of my head on concrete. Because the fall caused my left shoulder to separate, a quick trip to the emergency room was necessary.

An ER doctor yanked my shoulder back into place while I was anesthetized with Versed. It put my shoulder back on track. Versed is an amazing drug—it knocked me out for twenty minutes to jerk my arm back into its socket, but then I was completely conscious half an hour after taking it.

They told me that I talked about Buddhism a lot while I was out. I always liked Buddhism and have wondered if I was a Buddhist monk in a previous life. Their moderation, simplicity, and beliefs in the inherent impermanence of life have always resonated with me.

Another time, I tried to gather some papers I had dropped on the sidewalk in over one-hundred-degree heat in Phoenix, Arizona. That was not a wise thing to do, because MS makes my body heat-sensitive. I collapsed on the sidewalk and wet my pants. A Good Samaritan carried me to my car, so I could recover in the car's air conditioning. Fortunately, I was only two blocks from my house. I drove home, cleaned up, and meditated for twenty minutes, as is my habit.

The MS made me very heat sensitive. I became weak and dizzy when confronted with major heat. Getting out of my car into one-hundred-twenty-degree heat in my hot garage during the summer felt like someone wound up and punched me.

I remember collapsing on a hot day on the way to the parking lot next to my private practice office. An Arizona State University football player kindly carried me to my air-conditioned car. I now have a higher opinion of football players.

I eventually started to wear an ankle-foot cloth brace, as recommended by the neurologist monitoring my gradual downhill course. I was resistant at first but later conceded to the obvious conclusion that I needed the support for my right leg. I am right-handed, and the MS attacks always affected the right side of my body the most. I eventually needed a leg-length plastic brace for my right leg. I succumbed to driving my car with my left foot only.

The worst part of the MS was the necessity for me to be wheel-chaired through airports to the entrance of the airplane. I was a long-distance runner in high school, and this was torture. My wife tried to console me that at least we boarded the plane first.

There were visible acts of mercy that occurred spontaneously. Once a reservationist looked at me and my wife waiting for the plane and decided to give us first-class seats, without asking for them. She simply came up to us, took our tickets, and later returned to give us replacement tickets without telling us what she had done. We did not find out until later when we boarded the plane. God must hold a special place for human angels.

It is good to do good things. It is divine to do good things and remain anonymous. It also made me wonder how pathetic I must have looked in my wheelchair. On the other hand, people are always spontaneously doing kind things for my wife.

It must have something to do with her beautiful aura. She is always willing to ask for help. I avoid asking for help as I was well-schooled in rugged individualism.

After I graduated to using a plastic leg brace molded to my right leg, I did some physical therapy. I also worked out more regularly during the long-slow-slide into what seemed like coming oblivion. I decided it was time to get serious, which I will describe more later. The earlier you realize how dire your situation is, and how necessary it is to do the maximum you can to heal, the sooner you are likely to heal.

Do not wait too long to commit yourself. Take real action to get rid of this disease. Time is a luxury you cannot afford.

Chapter 7

Understanding Where the MS Originated—The Abuse

Early on I noticed, as many multiple sclerosis sufferers have, that stress worsened MS severely. I never realized how stressful flying someplace was. After taking a one-hour flight from Phoenix to Las Vegas where my in-laws lived, I would be exhausted, and sleep the rest of the day.

In my case, I thought my inability to tolerate stress came from underlying stress I carried within me from my childhood. It is hard to think well of yourself when you have been degraded to less than human by people close to you. As a child, I had a strong brother eight years older than me who took his frustrations out on me. I guess it was a stress reliever for him to pound on me.

It was like having a punching bag, only he got verbal feedback from the person he was assaulting—me. What I do not think he ever realized was that he was hurting himself as much as he was hurting me for no good reason. I did not want to be around when karma would later pay him a visit. What comes around, goes around, vigorously.

I had decisions to make regarding the MS, plus I had residual stress from my childhood. The biggest reason for that residual stress was the physical beatings my eldest brother delivered to me, which were unwarranted. He would beat me up on average once per week; however, the schedule was highly variable, depending upon how sadistic he happened to feel on any given day.

I tried to stay on his good side, which was futile. He once told me, "I would beat you even if you were Jesus-Christ perfect." This increased my feelings of hopelessness, despair, and anxiety to the point of paranoia. After all, what did I do to deserve this?

Alan was built like a world-class wrestler and could press 400 pounds. He was rated the best soldier in his fort during basic training. My second oldest brother, Greg, was four years older than me, and was similarly built. Both were amateur boxers at some point. No one in his right mind would want to get in a fight with either of them.

Greg participated in some of the beatings at Alan's command, but he clearly did not want to participate. I believe that he would not have participated in the beatings if not for the pressure of my oldest brother, whom I thought of as the Beast. I thought of my second oldest brother as the Accomplice. I guess I could refer to myself as the Target—it felt like a target was painted on my back.

Greg was heavyweight boxing champion of Fort Benning when he was in the military. The Accomplice once went through the floorboards of his motor home when he tried to deadlift 700 pounds on a barbell. At that time, they did not build mobile homes to withstand over 900 pounds of weight in one spot. When they were in the abusive stage, my brothers met all the criteria for white trash.

In many ways, I had a good relationship with Greg when Alan was not around. Greg away from Alan was a kind teacher who encouraged my progress in school. He regularly went running with me when I was training for long distances.

I know it may sound pathetic, but Greg never hit me in a way that would cause serious injury. He had redeeming features; however, all my brothers, including my younger brother, as will be seen later in this book, were fatally flawed. Between my flawed brothers and two angelic sisters, it is understandable that I naturally prefer women's empathy and compassion.

I once thought the elder brother, the sadistic Alan, was going to kill me. He cornered me in a shed and confronted me over some imaginary violations. He had a weak ego and was prone to see any random circumstance as a personal insult. He was a legend in his own mind. What was really frightening was that I knew that it did not matter what answers I gave him. He would make up a reason to vent and release his anger at the world for being born to my parents.

He began slugging me and hit me so hard in the abdomen that I almost lost consciousness. I subsequently was admitted to the hospital for surgery to repair the hernia he caused. I was all of ten years old. Why did I not tell my mother? I think I was bright enough to figure out that there would be no help, compassion, or justice from her sector of the universe.

My mother felt she needed my older brothers as workers on the farm. She also needed them as enforcers when she had to keep my bipolar father from making disastrous financial decisions. They gladly accepted their role as enforcers. That is probably what created a survivor's bond with my father—we faced a common enemy.

My mother was quite clever at making money with insurance. In those days, the early 1960s, you could have as many medical insurance policies on a child as you wished. The insurances did not coordinate with one another.

If she had two insurance policies on a child, one insurance company made payment to the doctor and/or hospital, and my mother legally pocketed the money given to her by the other insurance company. She was crafty like that. When my older brothers became eligible for the draft, she made sure they enlisted in the National Guard (much like the 2000 President George W. Bush did) to avoid being drafted and sent to Vietnam. The National Guard in those days was never sent overseas.

I became something of a major golden goose for our relatively poor family of eight children (four boys and four girls). My family reveled in their good fortune whenever I went to the hospital. I became known as "the ruptured rat" in my family's sick humor. Yes, that ruptured rat was a good investment insurance-wise. Alan made sure that investment produced.

I have always thought the stress of the beatings was a major contributor to the development of multiple sclerosis. I believe many factors typically combine to produce the MS syndrome. For me, the stress of the beatings created body memories, which resurfaced later in life when I was under stress.

The last time Alan beat me was when I was fourteen years old. My two older brothers hit, kicked, and chided me while I tried to lift fifty-pound hay bales from the ground to a moving hayrack. I weighed maybe a hundred pounds back then. The sadist drove the tractor while Greg was on the hayrack to receive my hay bale offerings.

I ran from side-to-side by the hayrack in ninety-degree heat, picking up single bales of hay. Alan stopped the tractor periodically, to beat me for not keeping up. When my father heard of this, he decided that he had had enough. No sympathy was forthcoming from my mother.

I never heard one word from my mother about what she thought of the beatings. I think she felt Alan and Greg were her army in her crusade against my bipolar father. She probably thought she could not handle the farm, my bipolar father, and the five children remaining of the original eight without my older brothers' superhuman strength.

My father called the county sheriff. They plea-bargained in a sense. No charges would be pressed if both of my older brothers left the farm. They both left and obtained prime employment plucking chickens.

I bet they were the best chicken-pluckers around. I must admit I developed a newfound appreciation for chickens. My feeling was "good riddance, and do not let the door hit your backside as you leave." I hoped nothing disastrous, calamitous, terrifying, or humiliating would happen to them. I did not want them to experience what I did. I would not treat any animal the way they treated me.

I later became a psychologist and had some interesting conversations with some empathic doctors. These doctors were clients I saw in psychotherapy with me as their therapist. One medical doctor noticed the correlation between childhood abuse and physical disabilities in her patients.

She shook her head and said, "Childhood abuse of people who later develop disabilities is so frequent. I used to be squeamish about asking people about childhood abuse, but now I ask disabled people if they were abused as children as a routine part of the initial exam. It is that frequent." She continued, "People who abuse children have no idea what they are causing."

You cannot imagine how much I agree with that statement. In my world, if you teach a child that he or she is hated, to some degree the child may come to hate himself or herself. Does hating yourself lead to the immune system attacking itself? It is not proven, but it is a reasonable possibility. It certainly seemed to be true in my case.

It took me some years to stop saying "I hate myself" when I was under stress. If you ever contract a chronic disease, and if you were taught to hate yourself, it feels like a certainty that self-hate increases the likelihood that your own immune system will attack you. Self-hate is an attacker you cannot defend against, because it is already inside.

Those of us who endure childhood abuse must at some point heal from that trauma if we want to live fully, regardless if we develop of chronic illness or not. Next I'll discuss my healer, who may have been God's way of apologizing for my brothers.

Chapter 8

Physical Therapy with Diana— Goddess of the Hunt

Somewhere around 2004, I decided to seek physical therapy. My insurance authorized standard physical therapy. The initial physical therapist did standard physical therapy in a standard way and obtained a standard MS patient result. In other words, it neither benefitted me nor had any effects—nothing really happened. The sessions met my expectations, but to get better, I knew I needed something beyond the average.

I realized I needed something different and strolled into 360 Physical Therapy in nearby Chandler, Arizona. The idea of this rehabilitation gym was they treated the whole body—thus the 360, standing for the circle as a symbol of completeness. Circles often represent the soul in dreams because they have no beginning and no end. I thought the place had a good vibe. It did. I met the goddess of physical therapy there.

The first physical therapist tested mostly my strength. I was very weak in the legs with poor balance. I had amazingly strong hands and could exert 120 pounds of pressure on a monitor I squeezed with one hand. Trainers have told me it must be due to something in my genetics. I immediately thought of my two older brothers, who could each bench press 400 pounds.

I had to get over the idea of throwing up at the thought that I share some characteristics genetically with them. It has been therapeutic for me to do things that are far removed and unexpected given "the farm" background. I prayed that some benevolent force would lead me to healing.

My prayers were soon answered. I was assigned a new physical therapist, Diana. She was an attractive woman who had recently received a practical doctorate in physical therapy. I thought I must have died and gone to heaven, because a blond angel stood before me. She would be the third angel in my life, after my two angel sisters. She would receive a lot of positive transference from the experiences I had with the prior angel sisters. She was knowledgeable, beautiful, and athletic, with an easy friendliness that met others halfway. Perfect.

In Roman mythology, Diana was the name of the Goddess of the Hunt and protector of women. Diana lived up to every aspect of that image. She was a classically trained ballet and jazz dancer. She was part of the University of Colorado halftime dance and drill squad. Diana was a certified yoga instructor. She was an independent, strong, and attractive physical therapist. I do not think she could have been named more appropriately.

Diana was smart, and I quickly learned to remember every word she said because they were invariably helpful. Diana would glance at me when I first entered and then proceed to tell me exactly what muscles were not working. She would then design an exercise, often of her own creation, that would specifically help the ailing muscles.

When we first met, I wore a brace on my right leg and used a cane. I would have a serious fall every week or two. I was right-handed, and the MS almost always attacked my right side. I was a mess. I was laying on a stretcher or massage table. She asked me to move my toes.

I replied, "I can move my left toes, but not my right toes."

Her commanding response was, "Okay, then move your left toes and think about moving your right toes."

I was happy to find someone who was capable of understanding. I finally found an encouraging physical therapist who was not afraid to push me even in the face of what I could not do. I like empathy. It is very different from making excuses as to why you will not try to do something because you have totally given up.

I was committed to doing my best despite the disability. I never stopped working. I continued to see fifteen, or up to twenty, clients per week even then. Working kept me going. Wanting to return full force to my private practice work was a big part of what motivated me to get better.

People often, in my view, make the mistake of conflating their disability with their identity. Multiple sclerosis was not going to define who I was. At least I would not go down without a fight. When you face a situation like this, it is not helpful to completely withdraw into yourself trying to find peace within. You do that at times simply to give yourself some space to recover, but you must be committed, in my view, to attacking the situation from a different perspective when you emerge from your temporary cocoon.

Jesus Christ said you must be reborn. Let me assure you that to beat a chronic illness, you must be reborn by pushing a process of aborting the parasitic illness. To stay a part of this world, you must be willing to fight for your independence and not make excuses for insisting upon doing so.

I was inspired to move my toes by Uma Thurman in the *Kill Bill* movie. In the movie, Uma is shot by a previous lover, Bill. The next scene shows her in the hospital paralyzed from the waist down. She is focusing on her toes and trying to get them to move. Getting that first little improvement is 90% of the battle. If you can get your body inspired to move, you have started to create a pathway that can be refined and improved upon, strengthened, as the body and brain dwells on the feedback it has received.

The movie was my inspiration in this situation. I would lay horizontally and try to move my toes for hours. As my method of focusing, I used "Kill Bill, Kill Bill" as my mantra. It was enlightening and almost frightening how well this visualization-mantra-ritual worked. There is greater plasticity to the nervous system than I ever imagined. The kingdom is truly within. At some point in 2005 to 2006, the physical therapy intersected with the steroid/Cytoxan treatments described later.

At one point, seeing that I was headed for a wheelchair, I went to the internet to find alternative treatments. I found an independent study that was used on six multiple sclerosis patients who were flat on their backs in the hospital. None of them could walk. They were expected to die.

They gave these six patients big bags of steroids for three days in a row. On the fourth day, they were given a shot of Cytoxan, which kills off part of your immune system. Because you are revved on steroids, you produce a modified immune system. It was hoped that the new immune system would be a kinder and gentler immune system that quit attacking your nerve fibers.

The treatment worked. Four of the six patients got up and walked. For someone like me, who had MS and was headed for a wheelchair, the effect of reading this study was like witnessing Jesus raising Lazarus from the dead.

I talked the great neurologist, Dr. Timothy Vollmer of the Barrow Neurological Institute in Phoenix, Arizona, into repeating the anecdotal study with me. He was of sufficient stature that the insurance company approved this experimental treatment. He had used the steroids individually with patients before. He had also used Cytoxan individually with patients. It was a new idea for him to use both drugs together.

They did this three days of steroids followed by a shot of Cytoxan every three to six months for two years, depending upon my reaction.

It worked. Not only did the treatments work, but the effect appears to be permanent, at least for me. (Other people may obtain different results depending on their unique biology and psychology.)

Diana noticed the switch in my levels of energy and improvements in muscle functioning immediately after I had the first set of steroids.

Diana insisted, "You have to exercise every day after the steroids. You can literally move muscles I have not really seen you move before. You have to come to physical therapy three times per week, and exercise the other days at home."

"Your wish is my command, oh, Genie of Physical Therapy," I joked.

She laughed and rolled her eyes. I was still a functioning male sexually. The multiple sclerosis had thankfully spared my libido. I was attracted to her, but more in a goddess-worshipping way than in a sexual way. She was on a pedestal and too holy for me to think of in that way.

My experience with steroids gave me a new perspective on the controversy regarding steroids in sports. It is true that steroids make you stronger. I felt 30% to 40% stronger after the three days of the big bags of 'roids, as I called them. However, the biggest change was in eye-hand coordination. I was middle-aged, wore glasses, and was sick, but I believed that if you pitched a fast ball to me, I could see the laces on the ball and was more likely to hit it.

Imagine the effect steroids would have on a young healthy athlete in his twenties! I now understood why so many baseball players had abused steroids. For me, it doubled or tripled eye-hand coordination— or at least it felt like it. My attitude after the three days of 'roids was *put me in the game, coach, I'll hit seventy home runs in a season.*

That must be what seventy home-run-hitter Barry Bonds thought (there were hearings on whether this Major League Baseball legend used steroids). We want to be kind to baseball players. The temptation to increase performance by that much by using steroids must have been overwhelming.

Diana then became aggressively supportive by encouraging me to do exercises I did not want to do. If there was one thing I learned from the farm and long-distance running, it was this: **KEEP PUTTING ONE FOOT AFTER ANOTHER**. That advice can get one through many of life's troubles. Being long-suffering and hunkering down and waiting for things to get better was a big part of the first twenty years of my life. I guess I did get some positive things from my mother.

Diana had me do the dreaded parallel bars. These were not parallel bars as one thinks of in gymnastics, but simply guardrails on each side of a person to help you walk—if you felt yourself falling, you could grab one or both wooden bars. I would walk sideways, one foot over the other, as I traveled between the waist-high bars that were bolted to the floor. These exercises were tiring and difficult for me.

It turned out that the hardest walking balance exercise to do was to place one foot directly in front of the other. The reason police test for intoxication by having a suspected drunk driver walk a straight line is because it is easily the most challenging way to balance your walk. After an hour of doing these types of walking/balancing exercises, I was exhausted.

It is interesting how walking in a balanced way is one of the most physically difficult things to do. It requires integration of the entire body with the brain. We take walking for granted because it is so common. Evolving from four to two legs was a major step in human evolution that freed the hands and increased forward vision and maneuverability. I often felt like I was trying to recapitulate evolution without looking like a monkey.

The other physical therapists would tease Diana because they noticed I always walked worse immediately after I left the gym than I did before I entered. When Diana pointed this out to me, I simply said,

"No pain, no gain." This playful and repeated statement was anathema to Diana.

As a certified yoga instructor, she lived by the idea that you did a yoga pose by trying to stretch just a little more than the previous day, but no more. My "no pain, no gain" statement was consistent with karate. I believe it was this mixture of yoga and karate attitudes, this mix of Yin and Yang, if you will, that helped produce the positive results. There is a time to relax and stretch and a time to break a building block in two. To everything there is a season . . .

It was enlightening to see the abilities severe multiple sclerosis takes away from you. I never realized how much balance is needed to walk. Walking through a dense and fast-moving crowd is especially difficult. One is constantly shifting weight from one leg to the other to make quick and often subtle corrections in direction of movement.

Some of the exercises were embarrassingly simple. One was to sit on a ball about three feet in diameter and balance myself. I bought a short stool to practice stepping up and stepping down. Steps were mostly "okay" going up. The main challenge was going down steps because one must land each foot on the next step with balance.

The radical steroid/Cytoxan treatments continued to improve my functioning. I was feeling 30% to 40% stronger after three days of big bags of steroids and my eye-hand coordination improved dramatically.

Diana and I sometimes looked at each other, and she would make statements like, "It's sort of a miracle, you know."

I would reply playfully with something like, "Oh, come on now, we both know there's no hope for this chronic disease. All you can do is slow the rate at which the ship is sinking."

Diana would smile and give me a brief glare.

I started doing some self-help yoga at home. I bought a book by Bikram Choudhury. He is from India, and his website is bikramyoga.com. His studios teach 26 yoga postures. This set of yoga postures is a comprehensive and doable schedule of yoga exercise. You do each posture twice, which takes about an hour or up to an hour and a half. I like it because it is a good sample of basic postures in yoga. It is a workout of stretching and meditating upon your body—what it can and cannot do.

I have tried doing half of the 26 poses on one day and then doing the remaining poses the next day, but that really doesn't work. The workout is constructed so that the exercises bend your body in all parts in all directions. There is a gestalt to doing the 26 poses in one set— you feel the beneficial relaxation after the stretches are exerted. I found it to be more beneficial to do the whole 26 poses in one set every other day.

It takes true commitment to follow this path since it takes an hour up to an hour and a half to complete all 26 postures twice. At one point, I was doing the complete set three or four times per week. At the same time, I was seeing Diana twice per week.

One week, when things really started to noticeably improve, Diana asked me a question, which went something like "How do you do that?" She had noticed that whatever we worked on improved. I explained that I did the exercises she devised for me in the bathroom. I explained that I visualized how the exercise was influencing the muscles as I did the exercises she gave me as part of my life routine.

To remind yourself to do yoga-like exercises, you must build them into your life. Every time I went into the bathroom, I did a yoga or yoga-like exercise. These types of exercises usually need no extra equipment and need little space to perform them. You would be amazed at how many times you walk into the bathroom during an average day. A lot of exercise can be accomplished following this routine.

I think the conscientious application of yoga and the yoga-like physical therapy exercises was a big factor in my recovery; however, I believe visualization gave the exercise an extra "kick." I came to realize that the exercises made me stronger, but there was more than that going on. Yoga is a meditation that occurs because of energy transmuted through the body.

I was always fond of Yogi Berra, the great baseball player, saying "ninety percent of the game is half mental." That means that forty-five of the variance of a person's performance is due to mental factors (.90 times .50 = .45, which is 45%). I agree with his basic point, but would assign different percentages, which probably underestimates the effect of the mind in the mind/body duality. Physical factors are usually more significant, but brainpower/visualization of what you are doing matters a lot.

What you learn when fighting a chronic disease is that there is no duality. As you have some success improving, you realize they are inextricably linked—you cannot help one without helping the other. If you damage one, you damage the other. That is both hopeful and frightening.

I am working toward not underestimating the mind's power—and knowing how much the mind can affect our life is both uplifting and frightening. Most people cannot take the responsibility. It is more than they can bear. We want to assign most of the responsibility to the god-awful circumstances in the world. Most people overestimate how much they can change others and underestimate how much they can change themselves.

You are not only making your muscles stronger when you exercise. I would estimate that doing physical exercise accounts for about 70% of improvement. The other 30% is a result, I believe, of the exercise strengthening the muscle-brain connection, literally the mind-body communication via our nerve fibers. This was especially important with multiple sclerosis because MS attacks the insulation (the myelin) covering the nerve conduction system.

This theory would explain why weight lifters who focus on their muscles gain more benefit than those who heft the barbells without thinking about it. Intense focus on what you are doing when exercising is using brain-cell-body-memory to make subtle adjustments that will benefit your body the most. Your subconscious and body is usually programmed to make movements in the most beneficial way, but we should focus intently until it becomes an automatic part of our body-brain memories.

It helped that in my workouts I was focused when doing the regimen of exercises. It helped that I wanted to impress Diana. Having someone neutral who is truly interested in your progress is a gift from God.

Chapter 9

The Psychology of How Abuse Contributes to Chronic Disease

Part of the reason I was abused was because I was different from my mother's family, who were mostly lower middle income workers who had problems with alcohol. I was more like my father's extended family, which included professors, civil engineers, public servants, and priests. My mother distinctly did everything she could to keep her children away from my father's family. My psychotherapist eventually intimated to me that she thought my father married below his social status. This chapter gives the background of what my life was like on the farm. Please consider it a case study of how abuse makes one a prime candidate to contract a chronic autoimmune disease.

In my worldview, one must know that physical punishment has future consequences for a child. Whatever theory of mental health you look at, eventually it gets back to the caretakers of the child as an important part of any person's psyche. Psychoanalytic theory assumes that the child introjects (internalizes) the experiences of childhood so strongly that it can literally be considered part of the brain. Thus, we have the father introject and the mother introject.

These introjects usually are composed of the biological parents, but not necessarily so. The child constructs the introjects based on her experiences. A child can construct these introjects from any caretaker or important figure in his life.

A kindly grandparent, aunt or uncle, older sibling, or significant older friend can be used to construct these introjects. That is why a supportive figure in the child's life, such as a compassionate grandmother or admirable uncle, may become the majority figure of one of the introjects. These introjects many times guide behavior and emotions as the person matures into adulthood. The super-survivor child can use various models to construct her own introjects.

The father introject tends to guide actions. The mother introject tends to guide emotions. This is not absolutely so, but it is usually the way things work out after thousands of years of culture. The brain uses the feminine and the masculine simply as code. The masculine identifies an action part of the mind. The feminine matches an emotional part of the psyche. The male/female dichotomy could just as well be the action/emotion duality of parts of the mind.

The introjects are often a default system for the individual person. When you are in a situation where you do not know what to do, the brain, like a computer, defaults to the learned mother and father introjects. If these introjects are good enough, the person at least has a behavioral or emotional response to the situation that may be better than no response at all. If the person grew up with good introjects, that is usually the case.

Negative introjects have the opposite effect. If a person has introjects so negative that they are toxic, the response proffered may cause self-harm. Thus, we can see why early childhood experiences tend to either improve or taint later life experiences.

Transference simply means that memories from the past affect the mind in the present. Transference is an amplifier. Stressful present experiences can be magnified exponentially by transference of previous abuse. The abuse has been internalized by the target and can be poisonously toxic when triggered by any stress that is somewhat like what the person experienced previously. Transference of the abuse means a stressor that echoes the childhood trauma leads to the adult (the child who experienced abuse now grown) getting a triple or quadruple whammy when the abusive transference is triggered by present stressful events.

The Jungians (followers of Dr. Carl Jung, who was the master of dream interpretation) put a lot of emphasis on "embodied emotion." The brain is not the only thing that remembers. Abusive or traumatic situations can become ingrained in the muscles, bones, and nerves, unless it can somehow be removed by psychotherapeutic or alternate therapies. I believe that energy therapies, like Reiki and massage, can help access and remove abusive ingrained damage to the body. The body as well as the mind is an avenue to potential healing.

Emotional experiences tend to be ingrained in the body where the damage occurred. These traumatic experiences are truly embodied. Traumatic abuse tends to make an indelible mark upon the body that the subconscious never forgets. I believe I was "set up," if you will, for chronic illness from the physical abuse I received as a child.

When stress attacks, it attacks the weak points of the body. Previous damage can weaken that point in the body in the future. These areas must be encouraged to return to health by exercise, nutrition, massage, energy work, rest and more. The mind can help by relaxing the body and freeing it from anxiety and depression. These maladies create tensions that weaken the body, especially previously targeted areas of the body.

It was massive medical intervention, physical therapy, alternate treatments, exercise, diet, and psychotherapy that turned things around for me. When you have a chronic, major-league, and in-your-face disease like multiple sclerosis, you no longer have the luxury to go with only Eastern or Western treatments if you want to turn the disease around. You must become a connoisseur of care beneficial to your organism.

I believe many people have died because they did not use all available treatments. MS is a complex conundrum. Many factors combine to produce the MS symptoms. By the time a major illness like multiple sclerosis is diagnosed, the patient is already desperately far behind the curve. To survive this assault on all aspects of your being, you need to throw any reasonable thing you possibly can at the invading illness.

Any good connection to universal energy and helpful angels, saints, spirits, or natural forces is an alliance to be cherished. Medical, physical, and psychological interventions are your front line, while alternative treatments are your supportive and logistical forces. Do not underestimate the importance of social support. People can often live or die depending upon whether they have at least one person who truly loves them. I had the advantage of having a loving wife and a good marriage.

The patient dramatically improves the odds of beating an illness if a legion of spiritual, physical, medical, and psychological treatments is used to unravel the disease and render it clawless. Developing a comprehensive approach is what this book is all about. I believe the methods used and the general philosophy espoused by this book are applicable to many chronic illnesses. ***Multiple Sclerosis Mission Remission*** is about my combination of modalities I created that worked for me to fight the illness while living with it. I believe we each have the power to create our own unique set of treatments that work synergistically together to maximize our well-being in the face of chronic illness. It is part of the adventure of life to discover what works for you. No one but you can create what works for you. I offer my story as a guide and hopefully an inspiration.

The remainder of this book will focus more on exercise, alternative, and psychological treatments. Ninety percent of the medical interventions have already been described. Remission, in my view, is brought about by emphasizing medical first, concurrent with appropriate alternative methods according to the condition and the abilities of the patient. These alternative treatment methods are brought on board as the patient can absorb them and make them part of his life.

The alternative methods described are a smorgasbord from which the reader can choose according to her needs. These mostly noninvasive, alternative methods can be used to fight against almost any major illness or cancer for health and quality of life.

Chapter 10

The Foundation of the Abuse

My family of eight children and my parents lived on a dairy farm in South Dakota. My father had bipolar disorder, beginning probably at about the age of 42, but it was not diagnosed until he was in his sixties. He had poor judgment, and many times was willing to sell cattle for pennies on the dollar. He would be manic and stay up for long hours before crashing into a long, melancholic depression.

He had a blank stare on his face and would slink off to sleep in a haystack, hayloft, or shed for hours or days. Relatives and friends often commented to me what a hard worker my father was when he was young. I guess you can get a lot done when you are young and manic before the disease progresses too far.

He and my mother fought nonstop. My mother concluded that he was just being a miserable human being. Part of my high school morning chores included keeping them from killing each other. Often these efforts were only partially successful, but it worked enough when I separated them because they both got along with me. They accepted my peacekeeping efforts. They were simply intent on hurting each other, and they had little animosity toward me.

My father never hit my mother. It was usually a case of him fending her off from hurting him. This happened once or twice per week. Once my mother gave my father second-degree burns by pouring nearly boiling water on him. I could not wait to go to college.

There was no awareness of mental health in my family. There was little awareness of mental illness in South Dakota at the time. This stubborn lack of awareness persisted despite my father's descent into bipolar disorder and in spite of my second oldest sister being hospitalized at the state psychiatric hospital in Yankton, South Dakota.

She initially was thought to be schizophrenic. A social worker later figured out that she had psychotic depression or bipolar disorder with psychotic features. My vote is for the latter. She was released from the state hospital and was supervised in Aberdeen, South Dakota, by a kind aunt. She was placed in a supervised independent living program in her own apartment.

Meanwhile, back at the ranch, in response to my parents' bickering, my eldest brother Alan was in the process of perfecting a sadistic personality disorder. He had only one testicle, which (I am told) does not affect sexual functioning. I always wondered if his sadism was an attempt to bolster his self-esteem and manhood threatened by this condition. Was he trying to prove he was a real man? He had twin girls with his wife. I think that finally reassured him of his virility and manhood, and he calmed down after he married and had children.

I was eight years younger than Alan. Like many in my father's family, I did well academically. My resemblance to my father turned out to be a curse in my family. Not that it was a curse in my mind. Despite my mother continually insinuating there was something wrong with my father's family, I was aware of only one paternal uncle being depressed, who was still successful. I think the comparison of my mother's family to my father's family was so lopsided that my mother felt they were haughty towards her. The truth was that she was trying to mend an inferiority complex.

My resemblance did not inspire my mother to be protective towards me. I believe my mother subconsciously ignored the physical and emotional abuse that rained down on me courtesy of my eldest brother. He was angry, and I was his primary outlet. This is not meant to minimize the physical abuse my father received from both older brothers. In my father's case, it was more the threat of physical violence—actual physical violence between my older brothers and my father was infrequent. When it did occur, it was pushing and shoving for the most part. In my father's case, my mother gave my older brothers unwavering support, if not encouragement, for their flirtation with violence perpetrated against him.

There was intense Oedipal competition for the affection of my mother between my father and Greg, the Accomplice. The Accomplice was trying to get much-sought-after praise from my mother. My father wanted to have a decent marital relationship with my mother. My mother decided sometime after the age of 45, when there was no longer any intimacy between my parents, to favor the Accomplice and the Beast. They were her minions. Given the situation of dealing with a bipolar man with poor judgment, perhaps it was forgivable.

The worst thing that can happen in the Oedipal complex is for the child to win. It set up the Accomplice Greg as a favored being viewed as superior to my father by my mother. The Beast received some favoritism from my father because he was the firstborn son. While both the Beast and the Accomplice became mother's henchmen to establish her rule over the farm and the family, I remember only the Accomplice physically attacking my father. With a few exceptions, serious injuries were mostly not involved. The aftermath of their fights was typically like a kid who lost a playground fight.

There was some grace granted by the Beast to our father for the honor of being designated the number one son by my father. Some images instilled by parents in a child have the effect of establishing a protective aura, which children avoid dethroning. When you physically attack a primary introject figure, like your father or mother or a primary caretaker, you might as well be hitting yourself.

When you hit one of your parents, you are also hitting the image of them that was implanted into your subconscious as a child. This image is an introject that you will carry through life. If you have any sense, you do not want to damage that introjected image.

The Beast mostly intimidated my father, while the Accomplice would physically attack him in much the way a brother might fight with another brother. My mother projected her subconscious hatred of my father for all to see, and my older brothers were quick to respond. The Goliath older sons were the power my mother actively sought and groomed.

This animus-possessed (power-seeking) woman, my mother, had the control for which she yearned with the two henchmen. The only power she had in the world economically had been established by my father's previous hard work when he was young. She was a sort of Midwestern Scarlett O'Hara who was not going to let anyone take her security away. As will be seen, she always did what she had to do to maintain control. This determination ultimately had disastrous consequences, as I will elaborate later.

I remember one of the few times the Accomplice went too far in his mother-approved attacks upon my father. It was a particularly vicious attack, which left my father cut and bruised and looking like he was just barely maintaining consciousness. He shuffled away into the twenty-degrees-below-zero snow and cold. When the disappearance reached two days, my mother, who probably had some form of undiagnosed mental disorder, became scared and worried. Like Scarlett O'Hara, she made plans to protect her farm, which she clung to like a security blanket.

She was not worried per se that my father might have been killed. No way would that alarm her, in and of itself. She was worried about the Accomplice doing jail time for manslaughter. She gathered me, the Accomplice, and my youngest brother Jeff around the all-important kitchen table. By God, she was going to make sure that everything she had invested in the farm was not taken away. She typically worked outside on the farm eight hours a day. She spent the rest of the day maintaining the house, meals, housework, groceries, paying bills, and so forth.

Gathered around the kitchen table, she began, "It looks like we might not find your father. God knows what happened to him. We all need to keep the story straight. He went off by himself and froze. That's all there is going to be to it." She knew keeping the story simple was the best strategy. I sat frozen to my chair, hoping my father had not frozen to death in a snowbank.

The Accomplice looked down at the floor with somber eyes. My four-years-younger brother, Jeff, the Child, was his usual alert self and fully complicit with this master plan. This reaction foretold what a negative factor he would eventually turn out to be in my life.

I was trying to figure out if my ears heard what they heard from my mother. For Jeff, if that was the way it was, that was the way it was. He knew his standing was high with my mother, and he had no desire to challenge her wishes.

My older brothers focused their wrath upon me and mostly gave my younger brother Jeff a pass. After all, Jeff's appearance, attitudes, and behavior totally matched the lineage on my mother's side of the family. Birds of a feather flock together.

My father eventually was found in a hayloft. My mother's reaction was a mixture of relief and disappointment. Relief that the Accomplice did not have to worry about going to prison. Disappointment that the husband she now regarded as her nemesis was still in her hair. She was not evil—she saw herself doing what needed to be done to keep the wheels of financial survival turning.

The Child, Jeff, learned a deep and valuable lesson from Mommy that day. He learned that serving my mother's interest resulted in unlimited support from her. It was not a lesson he would forget. It was a lesson he would use like a weapon later in life. I gave Jeff too much credit in thinking he was a decent human being. He was an intellectually and physically lazy snake who would later slither through my mother's will and steal 100% of the farm inheritance.

My mother mainly showed affection by praising us for work we accomplished on the farm. She never hugged us after the age of three. We mostly tried to impress her with how much fieldwork we did, with how many hay bales we stacked, or by completing some ever-needed cleanup job on the farm. We were all psychologically starving for some positive reinforcement from her. It was addictive. We were like emotional beggars beneath a dinner table trying to catch crumbs from a banquet. We never realized that no banquet was going on. My mother was emotionally starving also.

I remember the Beast and the Accomplice plowing fields all night in the dark by the light of the tractors. I believe they did this to receive the hallowed smile, claps, and praise from her. Looking back, I think I may be too hard on my mother. After all, I believe she probably had Asperger's syndrome, which is social autism. She had no friends and was socially inept. She had no understanding that social standing usually correlated with financial standing. If her theory of the world were correct, ditch diggers would be billionaires. It never dawned on her that a large contributor to wealth was relationships and social standing.

With Asperger's syndrome, the person often has average intelligence or above, but does not really understand or easily relate to people. They literally do not "get" people. There could be a relatively strong argument that my mother was suffering from, or at least had a high-functioning form of, Asperger's disorder. She had a sister who had profound autism and was intellectually disabled.

My mother was the second girl in her family, which included three daughters and three sons, to have a disorder on the autism spectrum. Her younger autistic sister literally spent her life sitting in one place, twirling and twisting pieces of paper. She was not capable in any sense of living independently. I never heard her speak a word. She received twenty-four-hour care from my maternal grandmother before my grandmother died. This autistic aunt lived her life with her parents until they died, and then she was transferred to an institution.

Mom had no—I mean nada, nothing, zilch—social relationships. She visited her parents occasionally. Her relatives sometimes came out to the farm to get out of the thriving metropolis of Watertown with its 15,000 residents. Watertown residents always thought they were on the verge of hitting it big, which never happened.

My mother once in later life admitted that she used the farm as her security blanket. The Child, Jeff, had a blanket when he was five that he carried everywhere, much to the growing embarrassment of my mother. She finally and cleverly disposed of it by cutting off about half an inch per day until it became so tiny that my brother threw it away in disgust. Little did I know that my brother would later subconsciously apply what was learned from the blanket addiction to his addiction to the farm.

Jeff would eventually carve the farm into tiny pieces, causing it to disappear. This act was quite a feat, considering that the farm was prime farmland located near the intersection of a major highway and an interstate. Commercially, the value of the land skyrocketed. My mother's security blanket, the farm, blossomed into wealth. Mom had no idea that she taught little Jeff to cut the farm bit by bit into pieces until it became worthless.

I want to take a break from the farm drama. I think it helps you understand me and where I come from, so it is necessary to include in the book; however, I prefer to focus on matters far afield from the abuse of my childhood and the Western medical approach that only took me so far in my autoimmune disease that resulted from that background. Let us delve into spirituality.

Chapter 11

Prayer

Most of what I know about prayer, angels, and saints came from my Catholic upbringing. I even have a paternal uncle, Father Bob, who was a priest who wrote articles for the *Catholic Register*. He led pilgrimages to Fatima, Portugal, where the Blessed Virgin Mary appeared to three children near the beginning of the twentieth century. I remember him holding me on his knee as a child and remarking that I would make a good priest. He may have thought I showed some intelligence and curiosity that would propel me to the higher realms. I thought about it. Being spiritually uplifted had to be better than living in dirt in South Dakota.

I attended the Immaculate Conception school until ninth grade. I always thought that name was demonstrative of how the Church felt about sex. Married Catholics were encouraged to have sex for procreation. Strict abstinence was the decree for the unmarried. Having children was vital to supply future brainwashed members of the Church. Birth control was frowned upon because it reduced the Church's growth. Very few Catholics, married or not, followed this misguided dictate.

I received all the sacraments to ensure my entrance into heaven. Nobody asked me if I wanted to receive them. It was the family's responsibility to make sure that everyone stayed in line in the relentless indoctrination executed by the Catholic Church, and what I am about to tell you may not be gospel, but it is the Word according to Steven Fox. In any case, like the *Course in Miracles*, which will be covered after talking about the Church, these beliefs and prayers helped me stand fast in the face of adversity and promoted my health.

I have arrived where many Catholics travel—to a field of ambivalence. I was given a solid structure that was reassuring amid the chaos of life. On the other hand, the areas of imagination and possibility that are necessarily stamped out might be too high a price to pay. I never did have children after being the seventh of eight children, and I think this is truly an accomplishment. I doubted my ability to parent given my introjects, and I did not want to inflict myself on a child.

The Church gave my family no instilled beliefs that stopped the abuse. On second thought, it was my father who stopped the abuse, and he was raised in a more strictly Catholic family than my mother's family. Maybe I have more to thank the Church for than I feel. The reader can see the mechanics of my ambivalence.

Let us first look at prayer. There are studies that support the efficacy of prayer in healing. One study (Byrd, 1993) involved 393 coronary-care patients in a San Francisco hospital ward who were randomly assigned to the control or to the treatment group. Church groups prayed for patients who were randomly assigned to the treatment group. Neither medical staff nor patients knew which patients were in the treatment group. The church prayer groups were simply given the lists of patients in the treatment group, and they were asked to pray for their health. Patients in the prayed-for treatment group did better. People who were prayed for were on ventilators less often, needed fewer antibiotics, and were less likely to have their lungs fill with fluids because their heart was not pumping efficiently. They were also less likely to die (this last result was favorable, but not statistically significant).

Larry Dossey in his 1994 book *Healing Words*, reviewed over a hundred studies. These studies gave support to the ideas that prayer can positively influence heart attacks, headaches, wounds, the size of goiters and tumors, leukemia white blood cell growth rate, etc. These studies are important, but are open to the criticism of the placebo effect and human suggestibility. But I offer this counterargument: if you are sick, how much do you care if you become healed because of a placebo effect? Getting better is real. The placebo effect amplifies the healing process.

Larry Dossey also wrote a book in 2014, *One Mind: How Our Individual Mind Is Part of a Greater Consciousness and Why It Matters,* which explains how it could be possible that intentions affect reality. Carl Jung previously and similarly postulated that we are all connected by a unitary "collective unconscious" that each person's individual subconscious feeds into. Perhaps this is how, for example, prayers can affect outcomes of health for another. Dossey's book offers evidence that supports this kind of paradigm shift that views all of human consciousness as being connected in a collective unconscious. Jung thought this collective unconscious explained why there are similarities among dreams, and as you will read later in the book, dreams have been an important component of my healing journey. The point is that we are all indeed connected, more so than we ever imagined (except for the Buddhists who have been aware of this phenomenon for millennia), and this connectedness is a source of healing for us all.

In many ways, and perhaps it is because of my background as a farmer, I prefer the evidence provided by Dossey's review involving plants, chicks, bacteria, mice, etc., because these organisms will not be subject to the placebo effect. For example, bacteria are unlikely to be suggestible. Examples of these studies included showing that volunteers using visualization techniques could stimulate or retard organisms' growth when they were fifteen miles away. It is impressive when corn seeds planted in a field, which were damaged by being soaked in salt water, grow better when prayed for, compared to damaged corn seed that were not prayed for. It seems very objective. It seems reasonable to me and others to assume that there is a significant connection among all living things.

The examples support the hypothesis that prayer works. They are interesting, but I believe they vastly underestimate the power of prayer. Life is not a double-blind randomized experiment. Prayer, by its very nature, is subjective and intimately involved with the human element of faith. Prayer, I believe, is likely to be more effective when reinforced by a friendship, blood relationship, or love connection.

I believe that if the person knows they are being prayed for (which is the usual situation in real life) the therapeutic effect is hugely magnified. It is more likely that the person will feel a healing energy, knowing that others are trying to connect with them in their distress. The placebo effect helps propel real healing and is a part of it.

In actual practice, the wise professional does everything possible to maximize the placebo or the faith effect, since it only adds to the benefits of treatment interventions. It is not placebo versus treatment effect so much as it is placebo + treatment = total effect. Yes, scientists are right to demand a positive effect from a treatment that is more than the placebo effect, but that does not deny that the placebo effect is virtually always a part of the total effect.

I have a specific way of praying that involves religious icons, saints, three different kinds of angels, and a master guide. Added to these are deceased friends, relatives, doctors, professors, and teachers. I constructed this method of praying over a period of years. It is based on universal principles of spiritual healing, but the unique entities who make up my prayer world are specific to my life. I believe this marriage of the universal and the specific in prayer is accessible and powerful for each of us. To be most effective, our prayer must tap into our deepest, unique self, while reaching out to that which connects us all as a whole.

My specific way of praying is described in more detail near the end of this book. Throughout the book, I touch upon all the various entities interwoven in my method of prayer. I come back to the topic of the universal power of spirituality in health and healing in future chapters, but for now let us return to some of the specifics of my unique, personal story as I strive to blend it with the various methods—mundane and sacred, Western and Eastern, mainstream and alternative—of fighting chronic illness.

Chapter 12

College Enlightenment

I was in heaven when I was in college. On the farm, it was a privilege to have the time to do homework and read. The desire to learn must come, to a large degree, from within the child for it to be effective. I lacked in that desire, but did enough to pass classes, until I was in the ninth grade. Mrs. Bea, my freshman algebra teacher, simply encouraged me with her faith that I could solve any word problem if I put my mind to it. I think encouragement is most effective when it points out to the child what he or she is good at. I was not encouraged at home. Rather, there was a reluctant acceptance that Steve could do school.

The Beast, Alan, unintentionally provided massive amounts of encouragement in my academic pursuits by doubting what I could do. Once, he was watching *The Bill Cosby Show* (this was the show before the more famous *Cosby Show* of the 1980s). Bill Cosby played an athletics coach who barely passed as also being a mathematics teacher. Alan brought me a problem that Cosby could not solve. Cosby hoped one of the brainy kids in class would somehow solve it without Cosby's instruction.

Alan brought the impossible problem to solve up to my second-floor lair, where I spent hours banging my head against the wall solving math problems. He left it with me triumphantly, certain there was no way I could solve it. After ten minutes, he asked if I could solve it, and I told him I needed more time. Ten minutes later, I gave him the solution, and, at his insistence, provided the proof that it was correct. The look on his face—priceless.

He never questioned my academic abilities after that incident. The funny thing is that I believe Alan was smart. He always knew what to do when there was a problem, usually more so than my father. To his credit, there were moments when Alan gave me a chore on the farm that he did not really expect I could successfully do. When I completed it, he would give me the high praise of begrudgingly admitting that I had done a better job than he thought I could. Alan fueled my desire to do things beyond what farm life expected me to do. College fulfilled this desire.

College helped me in more ways than even I ever expected. With the meal plan at college, I could eat as much as I wanted. There was a workout gym next to my dorm where I worked out every other day. On days I did not weightlift, I would go running five miles or more. I had time to take afternoon naps after staying up all night studying for a test. I went from 120 pounds and 5'10" to 180 pounds and 6'0". I was finally a force of nature that could be noticed. Girls approached me, but I did not know how to handle their attention. There was plenty of time to relax and ample time to grow intellectually and physically. My main thought was something like, "What a country!"

I was thrilled with the fact that I was in a place where abstract ideas had value. I tried computer programming, but found it too isolating. Computers back then could do very little compared to what computers were able to do twenty years later. I drifted into economics and business, but found it too boring.

I remember being in a business statistics course with tears coming to my eyes because the professor was boring me to death. I had already taken statistics through the college of arts and sciences, which was much more interesting. I was starting to demand more from myself and others intellectually.

I walked to the registrar's office one day at the University of South Dakota (USD) and signed up for all psychology and sociology courses. I graduated summa cum laude with a double major in psychology and sociology. (I was convinced that the only way this refugee from the farm was going to get anywhere was to get straight A's.) I was ready for a graduate clinical psychology program. USD was a respectable state school, and it even gets decent rankings from *US World News and Reports*. I liked the quiet, small town atmosphere where the college owned the tiny metropolis of Vermillion. It was a good place for me to study and prepare for graduate school.

If college was my heaven on earth, then graduate school was like finding nirvana. Clinical psychology concepts are initially difficult to integrate. Fortunately, the University of Montana graduate clinical psychology program integrated the research and concepts with applied clinical practice. It was based on the so-called Boulder (Colorado) model of teaching theoretical concepts mixed with clinical practice that the clinical psychology graduate program maintained at its student-based and surrounding community-serving clinic.

John (Jack) Watkins was the wise clinical director of the program. He died in 2012 at the age of 98. He wrote eleven books. He wrote his last book when he was 94 years old. He was a master hypnotist (he was once President of the American Hypnotic Association) who introduced me to psychoanalytic concepts.

Dr. Watkins was a kind and sincere man who knew everything should be mixed with compassion. He emphasized that "you do not train psychologists-in-training to be treaters of people by being beaters of people." He avoided much of the academic sadism prevalent in other research-oriented psychology graduate programs. Psychologists are not kind to one another—they are usually too competitive to consider that fellow psychologists have feelings too. It is for good reason that most psychology clinical programs encourage graduate students to attend therapy themselves at some point.

Prior to graduate school, I did an undergraduate assistantship at Norton State Hospital in Kansas, working with what was, in that day, called mental retardation patients (now intellectual disability) for six months. I did at least five assistantships during graduate school, which included working at the state prison two days per week for a year during my second year of graduate school. I was fortunate to win a scholarship that paid for the first year of graduate school.

Subsequent assistantships and work during graduate school involved a halfway house for incorrigible delinquents, a group home for the intellectually disabled, and working with a private practice group of psychologists. This latter assistantship included running therapy groups on the psychiatric ward of a general medical hospital, seeing individual clients, and performing psychological evaluations. I spent a summer in Boston at the West Roxbury Veterans Administration Hospital working with veterans with paralysis and head trauma. I also did an assistantship seeing clients at a university counseling center under the director's wife, who was a skilled psychoanalytic therapist. She was a deeply empathic psychoanalytic therapist who, like the director of our program, emphasized the therapeutic relationship in therapy.

While doing all this, I saw on average about five clients per week at the graduate clinical psychology clinic that catered to all residents of Missoula, Montana. The second through fourth years included practicums where we were supervised on the clients we treated. Frequently, we met with clients in pairs so that more advanced graduate students could show us how it was done. I needed the modeling and advice from the elder statesmen graduate students. I took a full load of classes always, except during the summer.

I took advice my second year in graduate school from a fourth-year graduate student, Nancy. We shared some clients together, and she always combined the right amount of empathic encouragement with clinical knowledge. She pointed out to me that there was a problem many stars of the program often had. The stars frequently sought to do outside extra credit and publication work, and neglected to complete their requirements to graduate. Her advice was to stick mainly with what had to be done, and confine star work to what little extra time I had. I walked the line on that one, because I wanted to be known. I wanted to be a star. There is little more intoxicating than seeing your own hard work in print.

I managed to eventually get my master's thesis, my dissertation, and my independent research project published in psychological journals. My GPA was somewhere close to 3.8. I was ready for the next dramatic change in my life—internship. Part of my attraction to clinical psychology was that it was completely unrelated to anything remotely connected to "the farm." After spending twenty-one years with dirt, cows, machines, manure, and corn, I wanted something completely unrelated to the concrete view of reality I was fed as a child. I relished my time in the world of academia, with matters of the head instead of the hands and back.

But we always take all of us with us, wherever we go, right? My spirituality was developing alongside my expertise in clinical psychology even if it was largely ignored during these years. That spirituality would come to the forefront as my body would eventually also take front and center in my life through the chaos of multiple sclerosis. Allow me to elaborate upon my spiritual beliefs.

Chapter 13

A Personal Angel Delivers Rules for Healing

Since reinvigorating my spiritual life after the diagnosis of multiple sclerosis, I frequently invoke the intercession of angels in my life. This is not angel-worship. God created angels before man and demoted them to serve man, which is why Satan rebelled. Their place in the celestial hierarchy was clearly defined, and it was below man's standing in relationship to God.

Angels are spiritually more powerful than man, and yet their primary purpose, if not their sole purpose, is to serve man. Satan did not have the humility to accept this arrangement. Pride indeed does go before a great fall. I believe angels primarily exist to help mankind carry out God's will. Man needs all the help heaven can offer.

I believe angels were involved in my healing. The most dramatic way I have experienced angels was through a dream my wife Debby had. She had this dream after I begged her to ask for a dream before she went to sleep. I was having my own dreams that would give me advice, but I wanted a "second opinion" from my wife, who was even more prone to have predictive dreams. I specifically requested that she have a dream about what I needed to do to heal from MS. Dreams usually respond best to specific requests.

She asked her subconscious for a dream about what methods would facilitate my healing the most. I am intuitive regarding dreams, while Debby is more generally intuitive and in touch with higher realms. I had high expectations. I was not disappointed. The next morning, I awoke to see my wife with this stunned look on her face.

I asked her, "What's wrong?"

She replied, "I just had the most amazing dream."

Before describing the dream, I need to give you some background. My wife had a secretary at work that she thought was like a human angel. The feeling was mutual. Kim was a very capable person who was socially gifted and would later go on to build a small real estate empire.

My wife and Kim communicated instantly on a level where words were often unnecessary. She doubtless knew Deborah in a previous life. There was a strange connection with me as well. Her husband and I had been in the same freshman introductory psychology class at the University of South Dakota at Slagle Hall. What were the chances of such a coincidence? I believe it is an example of synchronicity.

Kim frequently gave my wife gifts with cats on them. I believe Debby was a cat in a previous life. Her sensuality and cunning independence fortify my belief. My wife reciprocated by giving Kim, this beautiful and empathic secretary, gifts with angel representations, most notably a small crystal statue that we thought of as archangel Ariel. In the dream, Kim appeared to my wife as a radiant and glorious angel who sang four rules that I was to live by if I wanted to heal quickly. These rules were as follows:

1. Be nonjudgmental. This simple rule would accomplish 70% of the healing, as we waste immense amounts of energy being unnecessarily harsh and judgmental toward other people. Moreover, the energy we squander being judgmental of others has an exponential effect because we are usually five times more critical of ourselves than we are of others.

2. Show inner beauty. This pertained to my internal thoughts, attitudes, and intentions toward others. My wife remarked that I often do not accept that I have inner radiance. She said that

during this part she could see me in the background sarcastically quipping, "Oh, yeah, I have inner beauty." This one should be easy to accept, but in real life it is not. I had many clients who would have an easier time looking in a mirror when they were alone and saying, "I hate you," than they would have confidentially looking in the same mirror and saying, "I love you." Depressed people often find the first statement more compatible with what they have been told and believe about themselves.

3. Mirror the earth. This one was initially puzzling. I finally, with the help of my therapist, saw that it meant I should follow natural rhythms and cycles of the earth. Such rhythms would include going to bed at dusk and getting up near dawn, relaxing in natural places, listening to the ocean, being active in the sunshine, resting during rain, regularly resting after eating, etc.

4. Glorify the transfiguration. This mystical rule indicated that I would receive the most positive changes around that for which I was thankful and grateful. I was to sing praises to God, the universe, and myself for the hard-won changes I experienced. I thought that this rule particularly applied to changes in my body's functioning. The universe strongly rewards an attitude of gratitude. If you are not thankful, you can expect healing to slow and eventually stop. You know how it is when you suffer an ingrate you have previously tried to help—you decide that the ingrate will get no more help from you because he did not appreciate what you already offered with a desire to help.

I, of course, try to live by these rules. If you can follow the spirit of these rules, your life will be one in which you use energy wisely and stop wasting energy on emotions like resentment or anger. You also will avoid a lot of nonsense and increase your self-esteem and the quality of your time on earth.

Chapter 14

Go East, Young Man

After four years of graduate school, a psychologist is expected to complete a one-year internship. I was accepted into the psychology internship in Albany, New York, after wrangling with the determined, and later beloved, director of the internship. I was offered three different internships, but the only one I really wanted was in Albany, New York.

I tried to be clever when bargaining with each of the directors of the three internships. The supervising psychologist at the undergraduate internship I was doing with the intellectually disabled at the time, finally told me to simply tell each director what I wanted. He realized that I would not otherwise get what I desired, because the directors were unable to discern what I truly wanted. I needed to tell them clearly and honestly what I wanted, to get what I wanted. It was an important life lesson that I treasure.

A person can be too clever by half, as the English sometimes say, and thereby experience nothing but self-defeat. Things finally moved when I told them exactly what I wanted in no uncertain terms, even insisting upon it. I was ecstatic about getting this internship, and sang the song "New York! New York!" while driving all the way across the country.

Three facilities were located right next to each other in Albany, New York—a state psychiatric hospital, a city medical center hospital with a psychiatric ward, and a Veterans Administration Hospital. I spent four months at each facility. The effect was transformative—I saw patients from three different and important viewpoints. It was vital to my later private practice because I would see people who had been suicidal, had a major breakdown, or were in the military. Experiencing these major types of facilities and crises in mental health would be helpful in identifying when people were starting down the road to psychotic decompensation.

I later would see many people in private practice who had major depression, panic attacks, or Post Traumatic Stress Disorder (PTSD). My specialty in Attention Deficit Hyperactivity Disorder (ADHD) would come as a result of my private practice being near ASU. I experienced a personal tectonic shift in my life when I began my time in Albany, as my live-in girlfriend Cindy and I broke up after four glorious years of graduate school—right before I left for my internship.

Cindy was from Massachusetts and was an intellectual friend as well as a lover. I miss her if I think of her. My life would not have been changed to the degree it has been with Deborah, but Cindy and I were like two survivors on a raft in the ocean of graduate school knowledge.

I stayed out of relationships until the eighth month of my internship, when I was fortunate to meet my future wife, Deborah. I was lonely and drifting. Dr. Deborah Brogan, M.D., gave direction to both my personal and professional life. Deborah had few self-doubts, was the smartest person I had ever met, and was playful, fun, and kind. Everything about her was lovable. I had noticed her at a medical center Grand Rounds meeting, and her image was stuck in my brain before I knew anything about her.

Debby was legally blind and brilliant. She became legally blind because of type 1 insulin-necessary and primary diabetes, which she contracted when she was thirteen years old. The amazing thing about her was that you would not know how little she could see. She looked straight at you when she spoke. I frequently "forgot" that she was blind. The ophthalmologist I think realized how little I understood about her vision so I was asked to sit in on a vision exam. The first slide they showed was the huge E. She twisted her head at various angles and finally said after a long, long pause, "Is that an E?"

I never imagined that she had that much difficulty with her vision. I realized the reason she presented so well was because of her photographic memory. She often gave me directions when I was driving because she constructed a map in her mind from my naming the streets as I drove across Albany.

Debby often thought the stress of moving from her dear Los Angeles friends to Lincoln, Nebraska, as a teen was almost more than she could bear. Also, I have never met a sun-worshipping person to the degree that Debby was. Her worship of the closest star to earth was the reason we ultimately moved to Arizona. It was spiritually, personally, and professionally cleansing for her to move to the desert. Jesus met with Satan in the desert—I had no similar plans.

Debby was fast-tracked through college, spending only three years as an undergraduate because she was brilliant and because they knew she was likely to have visual problems due to the diabetes. She was valedictorian of her high school in Lincoln, Nebraska. After four years of medical school, she received her undergraduate degree concurrent with graduation from medical school. She subsequently did a four-year psychiatric residency in Albany, New York. I met her when I was on internship and she was in the third year of her psychiatric residency.

During my internship, another blast from the past thrust its way into my life. I did not know it, but I would be actively haunted by a sister. I was not close to her, but we always got along. Toward the end of my internship, I was rooming with an older psychology intern, in an apartment just across the street from the state hospital. Ken was 37 years old and one of the kindest human beings I would ever meet. He was in the wedding party when I married my wife Debby. At this point in the internship, which follows with the story of my sister's decompensation into psychosis, I was working on the E2 psychiatric crisis ward, which was filled with people who were either suicidal, psychotic, or both.

One late night the phone rang. I answered in my usual half-hypnotic stupor when awakening from an event-filled day on the psychiatric ward.

"Hello," I said.

The voice on the other end exclaimed, "Is this the Christian counselor I need?"

Initially trying to assess my spirituality, I soon recognized the voice as my third oldest sister, Kathy, who was around six years older than me. She was the third oldest sister and the fourth of the eight children, which included four boys and four girls. I was the third oldest boy and the seventh of eight children.

"Hey, Kathy, I'm not sure. What's happening?" I responded.

The voice on the other end timidly replied in a secretive, conspiratorial tone, "God told me there was a Christian counselor I should call."

I decided as a cafeteria-and-wobbling-Catholic-raised-partial-believer that I must be the Christian counselor she was seeking. I did not like the paranoid suspiciousness I heard. The way she sounded was similar to the way patients sound when they are going into a psychotic state on the psychiatric crisis ward. She was afraid, like most E2 patients are, of losing her mind.

"Kathy, what is wrong?" I proffered.

The desperate voice replied, "I feel I must get clear what is happening. Am I a good person?" she quizzed. Self-doubt virtually always precedes self-hate, which leads to major depression, suicide, or psychosis. All I could think was that this was not good.

"Kathy, you've been almost nothing but a good person," I stated as empathically as I could. This was like a therapy session, only my sister's mind was on the line and I knew it. What I was saying was not only therapeutically correct, but for me, was a verified fact.

"You would not lie to me, would you? I cannot take any more lies," she begged.

Telling her that she was a good person is one of the most truthful things I have ever said. She was an elementary school teacher in a small rural school in the Midwest. She took a year off in the middle of high school to stay home and work on the family farm before returning and graduating from high school. Three of the eight children did something similar, which was to stay at home for a year to get ourselves together and to help the farm and my parents' conflicted marriage.

The three children that stayed home for a year in my family were Kathy, Greg, and me. Kathy eventually became psychotic and died. Greg died in a trucking accident. I developed multiple sclerosis. I do not recommend that anyone delay education for a year to "get themselves together." In my experience, it does not work. You simply waste a year looking for something else, which may not exist. In all probability, you end up going back to school because opportunity is limited without it unless your family owns a business. Either that, or you get caught in a set of circumstances that does not allow you to return to school.

Kathy was a good mother to her two elementary-school-age sons. Her stress level was off the charts due to the machinations of her alcoholic husband. I believe that many of her conflicts probably had to do with his alcoholism. Gary was convinced of his own perfection. He stopped being a high school basketball coach and teacher sometime around his forties. He devoted his life thereafter to drinking and opining on the world's political situation. His two sons loved him and were dazzled by his narcissism.

"Kathy, are you taking any medication now?" I inquired.

"I'm seeing a counselor who referred me to a doctor who is prescribing Xanax," she said in a keep-it-secret voice. Xanax is a highly addictive anti-anxiety medication typically reserved for panic attacks. Many people and doctors recommend taking it on an as-needed basis, when a person feels a panic attack starting, to lessen the chances of dependency.

I implored her, "Kathy, I think you should go to an emergency room of a hospital to be admitted."

"What do you mean?" she said, taking my request as an insult.

"You are not feeling well, and are not thinking straight. You need to go to the hospital to rest and get your medication adjusted. Have you been having any thoughts of harming yourself?" I continued. I was in full psychiatric crisis mode now.

Surprised, she said, "Why yes, I have. How did you know?"

"When people get as anxious as you are, they just cannot see things clearly," I minimized. "You need some time to straighten things out in your life." The statistics and probabilities were tumbling through my head, telling me her survival was in danger.

She cautiously replied, "You wouldn't lie to me, would you? Because if you are not telling me the truth—"

"Kathy, this is as sincere as I have ever been," I said conclusively.

She uttered some words of half belief before saying goodbye.

Next were phone calls to our mother and to the counselor. Kathy reluctantly gave the phone number of the counselor to my mother. He was a social worker who surmised what seemed to be obvious—that "There might be an issue of alcohol abuse in the marriage." He meant well, and I know how hard it can be to say sound bites to relatives that they can rapidly assimilate, but I could not stop myself from thinking, "No kidding, Sherlock." My brother-in-law was in the running for being elected the town drunk.

My mother phoned me the next day in the afternoon to assure me that they finally found a hospital that admitted my sister. I felt relieved, hoping that a secure ward could contain and minimize her obsession with drinking water to cleanse herself, a kind of inner baptism if you will. That relief was unfounded—the bottom was ready to fall out. Early the next morning at around 4 a.m. the phone rang, and I answered in my usual zombie revival state.

"Steve, are you awake?" my mother said in her red-alert and anxious-but-trying-to-keep-it-together way.

"What's wrong?" I queried, knowing that she seldom calls unless the apocalypse drew nigh.

"Kathy died," she said.

"How?" I asked. We do not mince words in my family. We pride ourselves on sticking to cold hard facts even when experiencing stunned amazement or shock.

"She was drinking water all day. Way too much water. She had a delusion that she was evil and that the only way to cleanse herself was to keep drinking water. When she went to the hospital, they made her stop drinking water," she reasoned. This was the hopeful part, but then things went wrong.

"She somehow slipped into a bathroom before staff realized it. She stuck her mouth under a faucet and was taking in water when they found her. Her electrolytes were thrown off so severely that she died," my mother intoned. My mother was sad, but not hysterical. Never hysterical. This incident would become one on a list of a hundred tragedies in her life.

I took another hurried flight home over a weekend to see my sister hooked up to a ventilator, which was breathing a dead body. When it was confirmed that she was brain dead, the machine was shut off. Her alcoholic husband showed up in time to talk to some lawyers about suing the hospital. I talked to the lawyers about what was relevant. The hospital offered a settlement (I never heard the actual money figure) to her husband and two boys, who were around eight years old. The hospital also apologized. The case was closed. Tragedies like this have littered my life and led to my homespun spirituality. Let us look toward the spirits again.

Chapter 15

The Celestial Archangels

I see the first leader of the angels, Archangel Michael, as the most important. He is the archangel who led the angels in banishing Satan to hell. For that reason, second only to Jesus Christ himself, I see him as the embodiment of the heroic masculine. The heroic masculine, which is in all of us regardless of sex, is the action part of our minds (in dreams men tend to represent actions while women tend to represent emotions) that produces positive ways to change our lives.

In many ways, Michael is the soldier's angel, as good soldiers typically have a strong dose of the heroic masculine archetype in them—they are willing to die to protect loved ones or even cherished ideals. Think of him as the angelic protector who will see you through stormy times and onward to safety. I typically have prayed for help in being steadfast through hard times, to do what I need to do to heal, whether diet, exercise, meditation, or changing my life career-wise or residence-wise. Blue is often associated with this archangel. Blue is my favorite color.

Archangel Gabriel typically is a messenger in the Bible. I have often prayed to him to help me "get the message" of what God is sending me, whether a change in the course of the MS, or an actual message from someone I knew. One can frequently receive messages through strangers or mass media, especially if we are open to it. For example, a song may come on the radio, someone appears on the television, or a stranger says something that answers a question. I remember Eckhart Tolle, author of *The Power of Now*, saying much the same thing.

Most frequently for myself, platitudes that have worked in the past will resurface to guide me. Wisdom such as "Don't ever make someone regret they did a favor for you" (a direct quote from a wise doctor brother-in-law) can be invaluable. The acknowledgment, "Suffering a short-term loss is often necessary to make it to a long-term gain" (my observation, also made by many others) can be relationship-saving and financially wise. Injunctions to forgive others typically make more sense as we get older because forgiveness conserves so much personal energy that we can then use for positive purposes. The people we dislike are not worth the energy we waste hating them.

Archangel Gabriel is androgynous, as he sometimes looks in pictures, as if he could be either gender. I usually think of him with blond hair and a golden aura. I typically have prayed that he would help me recognize announcements of what was coming. I believe he was the angel who appeared to Mary to give her the message that she would be the mother of Jesus Christ, to prepare her for that role. Recognizing obvious signs of what is likely to happen is often more difficult because our biases interfere with discernment of truth.

Archangel Rafael is the angel of healing. He is obviously a primary angel in sending illness into remission. He is most often seen with a green aura. Green signals growth in dreams—it is the color of plants. He was a favorite of my wife's who would eventually have a pancreas-kidney transplant.

These archangels are the "Big Three" you need to help you heal. One is to protect, one is to transmit and recognize critical messages, and one is to heal. There are myriad other angels you can choose from to suit your needs. We will return to the spirits after a discussion of my return to civilization.

Chapter 16

Return to Civilization

I went back to the E2 psychiatric crisis ward in Albany, New York, after watching my sister become psychotic and die. A supervisor remarked to me that I seemed much more empathic. They never realized that this was the only way I could be with psychotic patients after the death of my psychotically depressed sister. She died of a rare psychiatric condition called polydipsia.

People with polydipsia inject themselves with massive amounts of water in a fruitless attempt to cleanse themselves psychologically. In this case, biblical images of people being cleansed with water is concretized in their mind and taken way too far. It makes sense in terms of what I now know about the subconscious. In dreams, water virtually always represents emotions. I believe she was mistakenly and concretely trying to cleanse herself of negative emotions.

I spent the summer after my internship rooming with a female psychiatric secretary friend, Mary, who was nearly forty years old. We spent the summer raising a garden together on land in the country that I rented. It produced wheelbarrows of some of the best tomatoes I have ever eaten. New York state is very lush and green. I only watered my garden once a year, on the Fourth of July. I guess I will always have a bit of the farmer in me after spending my first twenty years farming.

In my spare time, I was dating my future wife, Debby, and looking for a job. New York State decided to lay off many senior psychologists when I graduated. Positions for newcomer psychologists at the time were few and far between. A staff manager at a private medical hospital indicated that they would hire me sight unseen. I accepted the job as I was out of money. The only problem was that it was in western North Dakota in the small town of Dickinson. North Dakota's weather was ten degrees colder on average than was South Dakota's climate. I was reminded of this fact shortly after arriving.

I would be working on a psychiatric ward of a private medical hospital in Dickinson. At the time, North Dakota had mostly cows and beets and the fertile Red River Valley. Driving through western North Dakota, one could see frequent grasshopper oil wells. These oil wells were the precursors of the shale oil boom that dramatically reduced US dependence on foreign oil after 2010.

Of course, what I mainly remember about North Dakota was the cold. I did not previously think that forty below zero Fahrenheit with a thirty miles-per-hour wind was possible. After treating cold-shocked oil rig workers for that first winter, I became a believer that there was little holding North Dakota back from its seeming goal of attaining absolute zero. I do not have aversive memories of hot weather like the stinging memories of cold weather. I would rather take my chances with a heat stroke than deal with the constant threat of freezing to death or frostbite.

One winter day in that cold prairie town, the senior psychologist and I were staring at a windy blizzard through a window of the hospital. It was thirty degrees below zero at the time. The 50-something psychologist looked at the white icy haze that was overcoming the parking lot.

He remarked, "Why would anyone want to live in this cold, windy, barren place?"

"No kidding!" I exclaimed with unintended enthusiasm.

I visited Debby while she was visiting her parents in Lincoln, Nebraska. She always felt out of place in Nebraska after being forcibly transplanted from Los Angeles, California, when she was thirteen. Her paternal grandmother thought this trauma may have had something to do with her developing juvenile insulin-dependent diabetes when she was thirteen. To this day, many of her best friends are still in California. We would later make yearly sojourns to the same resort in San Diego, so she could visit her best friends who had migrated there.

I decided after doing my year in North Dakota that I had to get out of there, so I could join my beloved Debby in Albany, New York. I again obtained a job sight-unseen, which seems to be my modus operandi. Well, it was not totally sight unseen. The psychologist hiring me saw me present my dissertation research (which was later published in *Law and Human Behavior*) at grand rounds at Albany Medical Center during my internship.

I was hired by a psychologist who went through the same internship in Albany, New York, that I did. My job was to screen correctional officers for New York State for a year. We spent a lot of time visiting New York state prisons to talk to the correctional officers (guards) to understand what the job required in terms of personality and judgment. Oh, well, at least I would be near Debby. We married in 1985.

Shortly after our wedding, we both obtained jobs at the community mental health center in central Albany, which was also known as Green Street. That, of course, was the street it was located on. Debby worked with adults, while I worked primarily with children. People who knew us thought this arrangement was a fitting symmetry to our relationship.

I was half time on the children's treatment team and half time on the children's forensic team. I had been trained mainly with adults, although I had some experience with adolescents through my training. Before beginning my work with children, I assumed the issue of who children called "mom" or "dad" would be a big one for children of divorce. I found it was not an issue for the kids. It was an issue for the adults involved.

When I met with school-age clients long enough to know them well, I found that kids were quite clear regarding caretakers. Most kids called both their biological and stepparents "mom" and "dad," but clearly knew the differences. If they routinely did not call one of the four parties by a parental name, it was usually because they did not get along with them; or when the step-person came on the scene, the child was too old to become bonded to them. If you asked a long-term young client, he would tell you that he knew who the birth parents were, but he called stepparents by "mom" and "dad" because he was bonded to them. The younger, bonded stepchildren also wanted to acknowledge that a stepparent was a person who took care of them in a motherly or fatherly way. An additional factor was that these kids simply did not want to have to explain the situation to friends and others significant in their lives (teachers, coaches, and so forth).

The experienced psychologists and social workers urged me to treat kids like regular people and not try to always do the clinical routine with them. Occasionally I would forget this and start asking typical psychologist questions with a kid I was seeing. The kids would invariably look at me like, *Are you done now?* or *Do you feel better?* Then the client typically would give me a look like, *Can we get back to talking about the real stuff now?* In any case, therapy with children was completely different from therapy with adults.

Meeting with kids felt like a nice break from adult intellectualization. Kids usually give more of a straight story regarding feelings as their defenses are less developed—which can be a good thing. They do not even put scales measuring defensiveness on personality tests for children because they have proven to be unnecessary. Kids usually talk and react without censoring themselves. Remember, it was a child who noticed and finally said the obvious, that the emperor had no clothes.

Deborah and I deepened a friendship with a psychic social worker my wife knew, Claudia. She would later advise us by phone on which offices to rent in Arizona. The impressive thing about her was that she would make non-baseline predictions that became true. The office we had sublet from some therapist was splitting up. Deborah and I thought we had the opportunity to continue renting the office ourselves; however, another party, unbeknownst to us, had signed a lease already to rent the office once the original lease ended.

We explained the situation to Claudia and asked for advice. She answered that the people who were trying to lease the office underneath us, would, in fact, tear up the agreement and not lease the office. She stated that if we wanted to lease a different office we should look for one where there was a large pink blotch on the wall. She also thought the building needed to be near water. We generally believed in Claudia, but we did not want to risk our private practices upon it.

Two weeks before the lease ended, we looked for another office. The building we first looked at was a skyscraper with a large water fountain in front of it, and a large water fountain behind it. Okay, we thought, Claudia's condition about water being near the building had been met. We were shown three offices in the building. When the Realtor opened the door to the third office, we almost gasped. On the wall, directly in front of the opened door, was a large pink blotch. Someone obviously was trying out paint on the wall to see how it looked. We liked the office; all of Claudia's conditions had been met. We stayed in that building for ten years.

Dr. Carl Jung, a follower of Freud who broke away and established his own school of dream interpretation, would have called her predictions *synchronicity*, or meaningful coincidences. When two unrelated things happen in such a way that they seem related, it is time to pay attention because synchronicity is at work. I followed Jung's theory because I thought he took the most useful approach to dream interpretation, which focused mainly on the future, and not so much on the past.

Claudia recommended that I take karate to strengthen my aura. She thought it might help me feel more comfortable because it would encourage me to be more extroverted. I had a good kick, but I was as anxious as ever. Nevertheless, karate was a good workout and it made me more aware of how my physical presence affects others. Karate makes the karateka very aware of the aura we project and very much uses our spirit as a physical force to fend off opponents.

We need to discuss next how to connect this spirit with what I certainly needed, *A Course in Miracles*.

Chapter 17

A Course in Life

Somewhere close to the beginning of the new millennium, I started reading and applying *The Course in Miracles* to my life. I believe this book had a profound effect upon my perception of reality. The main point of the book is that things are not as they appear to be. When a person acquires a diagnosis of a chronic illness such as MS, he is very open to the idea that things in the world are not as they appear. He feels like a personal witness to something terrible that should never have happened.

The following text is frequently cited to summarize the main spirit of *The Course in Miracles*:

> I must have decided wrongly, because I am not at peace. I made the decision myself, but I can also decide otherwise. I want to decide otherwise, because I want to be at peace. I do not feel guilty, because the Holy Spirit will undo all the consequences of my wrong decision if I will let Him. I choose to let Him, by allowing Him to decide for God for me. (Chapter 5)

As can be seen, this book feels biblical. It is a brilliant blend of psychology and spirituality. A lot of it focuses on correctly seeing what is happening. It tries to clean our perceptions by helping us realize that our perceptions are deeply influenced by our past experiences. Cleaning the lens through which we view the world brings us peace and creates an atonement with God. If we make the correct decisions, we will be saved from guilt and negativity with the promise of being uplifted spiritually.

The course is not Pollyannaish and assures us that much of what we experience in the world is false: "This is an insane world, and do not underestimate the extent of its insanity" (Chapter 13). In many ways, its view is hardcore and unflinching: "This course is easy just because it makes no compromise. Yet it seems difficult to those who still believe that compromise is possible" (Chapter 23).

It puts responsibility for change and salvation not on others, the world or God, but on the individual: "you must realize that your hatred is in your mind and not outside it before you can get rid of it; and why you must get rid of it before you can perceive the world as it really is" (Chapter 12). It renews the promise that a big part of achieving peace will come through being nonjudgmental: "You have no idea of the tremendous release and deep peace that comes from meeting yourself and your brother totally without judgment" (Chapter 3). The key to discerning the real from the unreal is realizing that everything that is changeable or transient is unreal. Its viewpoint is that only what is immutable (unchangeable), or eternal, is real.

The idea is that one never fully realizes why she has certain reactions to certain situations. The profound point is that we never experience reality directly. We assign perceptions to experiences based partially or even mainly on previous experiences. We need to access the reality underlying life by recognizing what always remains true. This is no easy feat.

The book takes you on a yearlong journey of 365 sayings. Practicing them, by saying each one several times a day before going to the next one, will significantly help our ability to connect to the real. Here is a profound idea: I must realize that chronic disease is a lie I have allowed into my life. That is the bad news. The good news is that I can expel this changeable item from my life and overpower it with my immutable and eternal spirit. And you can too. Now that does not mean we stop using medication. We want to use our immutable spirit to resolutely cooperate with medical doctors. We need all the help we can get.

According to the book, we believe what we see is what we get. Actually, what we see is clouded by our perceptions to the point that we seldom see the rampant spirituality in the world. In my mind, this view is possible, considering that theoretical physicists assure us that it can be proved there are at least eleven dimensions plus time. We see three dimensions. It is said to all be happening here right now. There is much that our senses are missing.

It cannot be overestimated how encouraging it is to think that miracles happen regularly. When facing an impossible situation, it is hopeful to think impossible situations can be transformed because they are not real, because they are changeable. Multiple sclerosis is an impossible disease in need of a miraculous transformation. I was told it could not happen. It did happen. When the MS went into remission, I felt like I returned to my real eternal Self. Jung capitalized Self to indicate when he was talking about the soul.

One of the interesting ideas of the book is that there are no little miracles. A miracle is a miracle and evidence of the power of God. I was ready to free myself from the perception of multiple sclerosis, the big MS. It's easy to feel like you've let a cruel slave master into your life when you have multiple sclerosis. Remission is your Emancipation and Independence Day all in one, although it feels even better than that. As the great Martin Luther King said, "Free at last, free at last, thank God almighty, we are free at last!"

I always felt like MS was a huge mistake foisted upon me by the universe. My psychotherapist (from the early 1990s through the turn of the millennium and beyond) sometimes would try to get me to be at peace with the realization I would eventually end up in a wheelchair. She claimed I should accept this inevitability. I could only think to myself, "Fat chance, that." I put up with this singular fault of my therapist because she was quite insightful. Besides, my wife and my physical therapist knew I could do the impossible. That was all I needed.

I understood what she was trying to do. In her mode of thinking, by accepting that I had multiple sclerosis I could then fully realize the truth that I had it and could not ignore the effect it had upon my life.

But I wanted more. I wanted to be willing to accept that a miracle can be produced out of this situation with stubborn persistence and by realizing that the disease is not real. It is not God's will. It is God's challenge.

Chapter 18

The Family Mythology

The main thing Jungian psychotherapy did for me was to explode the family myth. Almost all of us are raised with the idea that our family has a certain, often unspoken, story or mythology to which each member of the family is expected to subscribe. Each person in the family fulfills a certain role to embody the complex family myth.

The consequences of a family member failing to accept the story or myth made up about the family can be severe. Nonbelievers are shunned or even excommunicated. The nonbelieving child is most frequently made the scapegoat of the family. Many times, the nonbelieving child who was made the scapegoat of the family seeks therapy to confirm that she is not crazy because she sees the world differently from the rest of the family.

My family's mythology went something like this:

1. My father was a miserable lowlife whose primary goal was to ruin my mother's life. This comes from no understanding of mental illness in South Dakota. Although my family was heavily impacted by bipolar disorder and psychotic depression, mental health treatment in my parents' minds amounted to the state hospital in Yankton, South Dakota. It is almost embarrassing to admit that my family was that out of touch. My father was finally diagnosed with bipolar disorder when he was in his sixties. He received the standard bipolar medications, which kept him stable. He still seemed depressed, but not as depressed, and he did not fly into manic episodes in

which he wanted to sell everything on the farm for two cents to close a "good deal" (for the other person, unfortunately).

2. My mother was a saint who completely sacrificed her life for the family. She came from a lower middle class family prone to alcoholism. I and some siblings thought she may have been sexually abused because she intimated, in those rare confidential times when we were amazed she was really communicating, that something may have happened sexually with a distant relative. She was uncomfortable enough and we did not want to interfere with her process, that it was always left vague with trusted children she confided in. It was interesting that she would never tell my three brothers anything like this—she had good enough judgment to realize that trust in them had to be limited. She told me and my sisters, because we were capable of being emotionally supportive. She focused on providing security for the family and herself. In my darkest moments, I sometimes thought her main subconscious motivation for having children was to supply workers for the dairy farm. Dairy farm work back then was labor-intensive. That was part of the motivation, but not the only motivation. The fact is, she was a strong person, screwed up by her family, who loved children and grandchildren.

3. My eldest sister, Valois, was an angel from heaven. This part of the mythology was true. She was fortunate to be the oldest so that she could leave the farm before things really fell apart with my parents. Her introjects consisted of a compassionate mother and an able and ambitious father.

4. My second oldest sister, Marion, was mentally ill and a danger to herself. This was a fact. She was strange throughout my childhood and finally was sent to the South Dakota State Hospital until some social worker figured out that she was

psychotically depressed and not schizophrenic. She was released and lived independently with some supervision.

5. My third oldest sister, Kathy, was a hard-working, good-natured, and practical woman who realistically evaluated the world. Kathy would later die of polydipsia due to psychotic depression. The first statement was true until the second statement happened. I never will know completely what led to her strange death. I think underlying psychotic depression led to the polydipsia. While I think the main factor in her decompensation was genetic, environmental factors such as her husband being an unemployed alcoholic could not have helped.

6. My eldest brother, Alan, was the number one enforcer of the family rules and leader of the troops. He, to his credit, mostly avoided conflict with my father. I think it was some leftover loyalty to my dad for being held in high regard as the eldest son. The funny thing is that I do not think this part of the family myth is false, but it was used to mask his abusive tendencies. He was able and smart, and most of his factual observations were true, which I guess makes it harder to dispel the negative things he made me repeat about myself while also singing his praises. How sick is that?

7. My second oldest brother, Greg, was a part of the Alan/Greg team whose work saved the farm. To a degree, this was true. They worked hard when they worked. This is one of a thousand reasons why Jeff later stealing 100% of the inheritance of the farm was ridiculous. Jeff, as the fortunate recipient of unconditional love from my mother and sisters, plotted to steal 100% of the farm, which he truly believed was rightfully and wholly his. He was helped in forming this tyrannical royal entitlement by my mother.

8. My sister Lauretta (I always called her Lolly) was an irresponsible social butterfly. She became Homecoming Queen of our high school and had an irrepressible, extroverted personality. My mother and Lolly never got along. They were truly opposites. Lolly would later become a registered nurse with a wonderful husband and family.

9. I was a reincarnation of my maternal grandfather. I did not look like him, did not think like him, had little relationship with him, and would manage my life the opposite of his. Family myths often defy reality. He later retired with a just-enough-to-scrimp-by lifestyle in a small old house in nearby Watertown, South Dakota (population 15,000 as it was then and as it is now). He was okay, which is why I did not defy the projection on me of his image. I supposedly was in his image because as I graduated from high school, I gave direction to the farm, which was usually followed with Jeff's approval. I think I did not react against it being said that I was like him because I was willing to accept any positive morsels offered by the family that would bolster my self-esteem rather than tear it down.

10. My younger brother Jeff made magic happen through his magnetic and overwhelming charisma. He would be the destruction of any wealth created from the farm. To my mother, he was a magician who made wonderful things appear. To me, he is simply the Child. He turned out to be the Child who liked to play with fire.

Chapter 19

Reiki to the Rescue

When Debby and I first came to Arizona, a female psychologist named Barbara, who was fascinated with alternative views of reality, recommended that we learn Reiki. We contacted the recommended turban-wearing Sikhs. I did not know what to make of the two Sikhs at first. Sangeet was a woman who was a powerful Reiki master. Her husband, Hari Nam, assisted in the training of this ancient art. I was skeptical until I was a recipient of Sangeet's life force of Reiki. Her power and abilities in exerting a physical force of warmth through her hands was unbelievable. I felt it was uncanny and had no explanation for it.

In Reiki, the recipient lies face up on a carpet or mat while the Reiki master, Sangeet in this case, holds her hands about six to nine inches from areas believed to be critical for functioning. All the main chakra areas are Reiki-ed. I dutifully laid down, closed my eyes, and expected to feel nothing.

The first time, after fifteen minutes or so, I felt like someone was standing on my abdomen. I opened my eyes to see Sangeet focusing on me intensely with her hands about half a foot from my stomach. My skepticism declined rapidly. How could she exert that much physical force? I was trained in hypnosis and did not feel like she put me in a trance where I would have trouble discerning what was going on.

When doing Reiki, the healer focuses on feeling heat from the patient's body. This is not hard. It is surprisingly easily detected. As Deepak Chopra says, "One does not have to go looking for God. God is unavoidable." I think Reiki is part of the old practice of laying on of hands. It seems different in that it is teachable, and directions can be given as to how to do it. This contrasts with the style of laying on of hands where it simply is assumed that with enough faith God intervenes and a miracle of healing occurs.

An interesting fact is that parts of the body in need of healing generate heat, as we observe with illness or infection. The Reiki healer can feel heat going out from the hands. To experience a small part of this, simply take your right hand and hold it four to six inches palm-down above your left hand which should be held palm up. One can feel a flow of energy between the two hands. The body is motivated to heal and sends heat energy to heal.

In the case of fever and infection, the danger is that the body will overwhelm itself with the chi, or heat energy. Reiki administers a flow of energy that is naturally regulated between the healer and patient. The heat energy is administered at the ideal temperature to help the patient. For this reason, it is important that the healer be in a state of homeostatic equilibrium so that the optimal healing energy is transferred to the patient without overtaxing his major organ systems.

At the first and most basic level, the healer focuses on the flow of energy through the hands while repeating a mantra and visualizing the design of a specific ancient symbol. The first symbol is the Reiki Power Symbol. There are other advanced symbols meant to straighten, improve, and increase the range of the Reiki energy being delivered.

I cannot divulge the mantras nor draw the symbols for you. I have taken a vow not to reveal this information to non-initiates of Reiki. The ancient masters who taught Reiki to initiates would draw the symbols in the sand, and then erase them when the lesson was over.

Persons interested in Reiki should learn it from a master Reiki teacher. Their world is something different and powerful. To this day, I return when needed to Sangeet, my master Reiki teacher, when I am having physical problems. I do Reiki on my wife Debby, and we both feel the Reiki energy flowing through me is stronger than ever.

I am always amazed at how powerful the Reiki force flowing through Sangeet is. She is 72 years old, and her ability to conduct the Reiki force is even more powerful than when I first met her. When she is focusing on my head, it feels like an electrical field is at work. Practice does make perfect.

It is important to know that this energy is positive energy coming from the universe and not from the master or the healer. The field of electricity-like energy is merely flowing through the master who has perfected transferring the energy to the recipient. It must come from the universe, as the master would soon be depleted of vitality if it were not.

We met with Sangeet and Hari Nam for three weekends to learn the four basic signs of Reiki. With these four symbols, the trainee was a third-degree Reiki practitioner. Months of practice followed each weekend.

Several times, we met with the public to practice Reiki skills on volunteers. Recipients were usually thankful and enjoyed the experience. The next level was to make Reiki a way of life and become a master after years of practice. Reiki was used in my healing, as my wife was a powerful third-degree practitioner. In my experience, people who are intuitive tend to be powerful Reiki practitioners.

Chapter 20

Synchronicity, Reiki, and the Flash of Light

In 1998, Deborah became the first pancreas-kidney transplant in Arizona. The circumstances, meaningful coincidences, and synchronicity that accompanied and followed that transplant are amazing. Dr. Fabrega was an unusual surgeon, in that he talked and explained everything. He was willing to meet the patient halfway on medical decisions about what procedures, surgeries, and medications would be employed. My wife talked to him for half an hour and was convinced that he was heaven-sent. There were many reasons for this belief.

That Deborah was the first pancreas-kidney transplant in Arizona was a surprise to us. We thought Arizona would be more advanced in medical procedures, but it turned out that the Midwest is usually far ahead of the rest of the country in doing transplants. I believe the reason for this is the prevalence of agriculture programs in the colleges and universities in the Midwest. The test population for new transplant procedures is always animals. In the Midwest, there is a plethora of captive populations of animals at the universities near medical schools on which to try life-saving transplant surgeries. We owe much to animals and need to be more kind in sharing the earth with animals and be grateful for and protective of their special place on earth.

The doctor that did her transplant, Dr. Fabrega, came from Iowa City, Iowa. The hospital where he previously worked was the hospital where Debby was born. He came to Phoenix just two weeks before performing the transplant surgery on Debby, which was performed on an emergency basis. Those meaningful circumstances were the workings of synchronicity.

Even the way her surgery was delayed was a miracle. She saw a nephrologist for years who monitored her lab tests, which were god-awful, but he never did anything. The leader of the group practice finally demanded to look at the lab tests after Debby was in crisis. He decided that she needed to go for dialysis immediately. After years of delay, the leader of the group practice decided that she needed emergency surgery to do dialysis to save her life.

Why had surgical intervention been put off so long? It was because her nephrologist was a well-meaning idiot. Debby had this peculiar quality of always appearing healthy regardless of how bad the lab tests were. He actually got into the habit of ignoring lab tests because it did not agree with the healthy vision of Debby he had in his mind. When we asked our friendly psychic Claudia about Debby's health, she stated that her guides simply blocked any visions into Debby's health and indicated that was not an area to question.

In short, the guide's advice to Claudia was, "DON'T GO THERE!"

We later understood that it was vital that the nephrologist was an idiot regarding Debby, so that intervention could be delayed until she had the right donor and the right surgeon in the right place at the right time. In addition, during those extra years granted by the good doctor's non-observation of the obvious, better anti-rejection drugs were invented that were much better at preventing pancreas rejection, such as Cellcept. During that time, the pancreas transplant success rate went from 50% to 80% because of the better anti-rejection drugs.

Because she needed dialysis immediately, there was no time for surgery to build a "port" on one of her forearms that typically was installed before dialysis was started. They simply made a temporary dialysis entry point on her chest near her heart. It was a good thing that they used this temporary arrangement because she was on dialysis for only two weeks.

There was the usual hassle with insurance to approve the future transplants. In anticipation, Dr. Fabrega had her do a heart catheterization. He wanted to make sure her heart was strong. He noted that frequently it was the heart that determined success. That is true physically and emotionally in my world. The only thing that remained was to find a donor, which had to be a cadaver, because living people cannot donate a pancreas; we only have one.

The donor was an eighteen-year-old man who died from meningitis. Debby was at the top of the transplant list for several reasons:

1. She was the first on the pancreas transplant list because there was no pancreas list in Arizona prior to this surgeon, Dr. Fabrega, transferring to Phoenix.

2. She already and recently had a heart catheterization to check out the strength of her heart (whether the patient makes it through the transplant or not often boils down to the strength of the heart).

3. They needed an Arizona recipient who was ready for transplant now or they would have to send the harvested organs to California.

She received the fateful phone call from the hospital telling her that the insurance approved the transplants and ("Are you sitting?") that she should come to the hospital immediately because they had a donor. A Reiki practitioner who had been taught at high levels, we will say his name was Mark, happened to see Debby immediately after she received the phone call to come to the hospital to receive the transplants. Mark came up to me in our private practice office after he saw Debby leave for the hospital. He had a wide-eyed look of amazement on his face.

Alarmed, I asked, "What's wrong?"

Mark replied, "I just saw Dr. Brogan surrounded by blinding white light."

He was shocked and surprised. I was not. I had never known a sicker healthy person or a healthier sick person than Debby. I could never decide which it was. Living with Debby was a series of transcendent experiences.

For example, after the transplant, which completely cured her of Type 1 diabetes, she became medically intuitive. She could see inside the bodies of people who asked her to look. She could accurately tell a pregnant woman the sex of the baby prior to medical testing. She once was able to see that her pregnant friend had triplets in her womb before ultrasound confirmed it. It is not proper protocol to look intuitively unless the recipient gives the intuitive permission to do so. The celestial realm has rules of confidentiality also—most meaningful relationships do.

Medical tests such as CT scans on Debby's own body confirmed what she saw from her own intuitive searching. Once the CT scan diverged from Deborah's opinion. After they followed my wife's recommendation to increase the magnification of the scan, they saw what she saw in the same location. Doctors stopped doubting her self-report regarding her own bodily-physical intuitions.

It was remarkable that, for two or three years after the transplant, many of Deborah's personal tastes in food changed to be more like what you would expect from an eighteen-year-old man. She was almost vegan prior to the surgery, although she would do "social chicken." After the transplant from her eighteen-year-old male donor, she wanted some form of meat and potatoes each day. She started to snack on dry Cheerios. Her diet looked like what you would expect from an eighteen-year-old teenager. I sometimes joked that if she started to drink beer, watch Monday night football, and fart—it was time for divorce.

We think that what happened is that body cell memory from the transplanted organs created cravings for previously familiar foods. The fact that the pancreas is heavily involved with digestion strengthens that point of view. In any case, these cravings gradually disappeared. I sometimes wondered if the pancreas experienced a mix of yearning and relief because where once there was sugar aplenty, suddenly there was much less demand to digest sugar from 97-pound Debby than from a male teenager. For now, I need to return to giving more background on what led to our journey from upstate New York to our personal oasis of healing in the desert of Phoenix, Arizona.

Chapter 21

Here Comes the Sun and the Kundalini of Yoga

When we lived in Albany, New York, the weather was almost permanently cloudy. My wife complained that it was hopeless to go to the beach because of the clouds. I came to understand how subjective weather reports are. Often when the radio assured us that it was sunny, it was actually partly cloudy by Phoenix standards. It was the darkest part of Hades by my wife's standards.

I realized that Debby and I needed some additional physical activity. She was getting little exercise and mostly mourning the loss of her access to the beach as a child. I started taping television shows that featured a half hour of yoga. It was about the right amount of time for Debby. It was about the right level of challenge for Debby. The yoga instructor said she was a "Georgia peach" and was "Nifty Fifty."

Debby took to the practice of yoga with unexpected fervor. I would come into the living room sometimes to see her doing the same yoga pose as the videotaped instructor. One of them was doing the pose as a model of perfection. The instructor didn't look half-bad either. I am not exaggerating.

The yoga was a temporary fix for my wife's yearning for activity even though it was not basked in sunshine. Her health decreased when she was not able to experience the sun for extended periods of time. Sunshine was almost as necessary for Debby's health as water is for other people's physical health—well, at least as necessary for her as protein is for other people.

One June and July in 1987, my wife was furious that we could not go on planned excursions to the beach because it was cloudy. This happened eight weekends in a row. It was the beginning of a frequent refrain from Debby: "You have to get me out of here. My body cannot take this weather!"

I believed her. Albany doctors, in that negative healing mode doctors assume so that they do not raise the patient's expectations and get sued, assured me that she would die sometime in her thirties. Since Debby was not kidding about the necessity of sunshine for her physical health, I decided it was time for decisive action. I am not often decisive, but when I am, my world spins to a new place.

I looked at a map of the USA for the sunniest place in the country. Phoenix, Arizona looked like it was the place. I subsequently learned that days Phoenix called "partly cloudy" would have been celebrated as "blazing sunshine" in Albany. There are 69 days of sunny weather in Albany on average per year. There are 111 "partly sunny" days in Albany per year on average. These facts mean that there are only 180 days with some sun during the entire year in Albany on average.

That means more than half of the days of the year in Albany are cloudy. Eight-two percent of the year in Phoenix is sunny—299 days of glorious sunshine with low humidity! The two weeks of 120-degree Fahrenheit weather during June or July each summer only affects those of us who are in the sun away from air conditioning or who need to depart on an airplane. That's right. It actually gets too hot for some smaller jets to safely take off from the Phoenix airport during some days in June or July.

I saw an ad for a psychiatrist at the ASU Student Health Center. ASU was one of the largest universities in the country. I insisted that she apply for the job, as she always had wanted to work at a university student health center. We sold the house near Albany that we had lived in for only ten months and headed for the Southwest. It was too bad in a way. I will never forget and miss the sound of our twenty-pound cat rumbling through the upstairs crawlspace of the Cape-Cod-style house we briefly owned in Albany, New York.

In addition to teaching Reiki, our outstanding Sikhs also knew Kundalini Yoga. Of Sangeet and Hari Nam, Hari Nam was our main instructor. The main idea of Kundalini yoga is that it releases the serpent of energy at the base of the spine. Yogi Bhajan popularized Kundalini, the "yoga of awareness." He brought it to the United States from India in the 1960s. Sangeet was a friend of Yogi Bhajan, and we would get to meet him.

In Kundalini yoga, the main emphasis is on breathing. The Kundalini exercises are basically synchronized breathing. For example, Breath of Fire is all about continuous breathing. One kneels and sits back on the feet while bellows breathing. You then take in quick and shallow inhalations while exhalations are fired with short and rapid bursts of forced air. It was a legend that you could not die while performing breath of fire.

A concept in Kundalini is that each person is destined to take a certain number of breaths in life; however, one does not shorten his life with breath of fire because each episode of a breath of fire session counts as one breath. The legend that one could not die while doing breath of fire may not be practical in the sense of adding days to your life, but it could extend your life for a few minutes while waiting for the ambulance or loved ones to arrive. I made a personal note to keep this technique in mind if I was near the end and needed to extend my life for a minute or two. Maybe I would get that apology from the Beast in my final seconds of life. No, that is unlikely to happen, even over my dead body.

Kundalini yoga is the only type of yoga considered to be potentially dangerous. Dr. Carl Jung thought that Eastern techniques had potential danger because they can release too much energy, more energy than the person's mind or psyche could handle. I am a strong believer in the concept that anything strong enough to heal probably has equal ability to do harm if handled inappropriately.

Kundalini yoga is all about releasing energy. Doing it too intensely can be harmful, so the initiate is well advised to learn Kundalini yoga from an experienced yogi. The safer type of yoga is Hawthorne yoga.

Hawthorne yoga is more what I would call exercise yoga. You do the pose twice each day for an extended pause, which virtually always involves balance and stretching, but there is some weight-bearing in the sense of standing on one leg or using the arms to stretch and support, and sometimes lift, the body. I felt the more actively physical Hawthorne yoga was probably a better fit for me.

Bikram's Beginning Yoga Class by Bikram Choudhury is an excellent yoga book with twenty-six common yoga poses. There are many Bikram yoga studios in the United States. These poses are well known, such as the Standing Bow, Camel, and Child poses. There is a purpose to the order in which the poses are performed as one generally stretches in the opposite or different direction with your body compared to the previous pose. It feels like a total workout of the whole body that is a sort of thoughtful body meditation.

One does each pose only twice. The poses are best performed in the order presented by Bikram because they bend the spinal column in alternate ways. One only goes as far as is possible without feeling pain. Never fear, the person almost invariably comes closer and closer to doing the pose correctly with daily practice. With faithful practice and concentration, you will see slow but certain improvement that rejuvenates your body and attitude.

Doing yoga is a commitment. I typically need an hour and a half session to complete all twenty-six poses twice. I experimented with doing half one day and half the next day and found it unsatisfying. There is something about doing the whole routine at once that seems like a holistic necessity. My wife was skilled at mastering the routine by doing fifteen-minute drills in front of the television on a daily basis. To each his own. You must find the rhythm and technique that fits your biology and temperament.

Chapter 22

The Agony of Defeat

Next to me, my younger brother Jeff is probably the most difficult to explain. Being the baby of the family was true for Jeff, literally and figuratively. Having four beautiful sisters and my mother who showered him with adoration constellated much of his personality. One would think that such attention would have resulted in some positive characteristics, which it has—he is mostly immune to major depression or panic disorder.

On the other hand, the effect of such attention depends on how the individual receives it. How it affects the person depends on the recipient's basic temperament. Jeff took it to mean that he was king and deserved everything. He basically became a narcissist.

He had no self-esteem issues and never thought he received more than he deserved. In fact, he believed he deserved more than he received. This lack of insight into the needs of others would be the source of his early success and the cause of his ultimate defeat. He became impulsive and reckless, failing to recognize there are consequences for irresponsible behavior.

While I was in therapy during most of the 1990s after I contracted multiple sclerosis, Jeff sold the dairy cattle of the farm. He rented the land out. He sold some farmland so that a gas station and motel could be built next to an interstate. All the dreams of the farm someday becoming valuable were coming true. But wait, there's more.

He helped manage the motel for a while and later ran his own carpet cleaning business. He subsequently obtained a liquor license. He also somehow managed to get the rights so that gambling could be enjoyed in his bar. The carpet business was transformed into a casino, which was named Foxy's.

Jeff had no idea, and did not care about, the shadow elements he was allowing into his life with gambling. I never set foot in South Dakota to witness what recklessness could accomplish in prosperous economic times. I am so glad I never beheld the travesty that would ultimately lead to Jeff's economic demise.

By 2008, he was flying high. His grandiosity and hyperactivity, punctuated by bouts of irritability, would allow the entrance of malignant possibilities. Like Icarus in Greek mythology, he would fly too close to the sun, melting his wings so that he crashed into reality. I came to understand the complex proverb, "A beggar mounted races his steed." He had increasing financial horsepower, but had not cultivated the wisdom to manage it. The economic horse he rode was recklessly raced.

And he was racing toward disaster. A more intense disaster would follow the initial disaster. It turned out that his first wife, Connie, had a gambling problem that was out of control. They went to therapy, and my brother claimed Connie blamed him for her addiction.

I remember having to drag Jeff away from carnival games when he was a kid. He resisted leaving situations where he was losing money. Just as he was unable to walk away from rigged carnival games, he was unable to walk away from poor deals he had made.

They eventually divorced. She now would receive half of the thriving little casino for bringing it to financial ruin. In her sadness, I believe Connie must have received $200,000 or more in the divorce settlement. Sometimes what looks like a disaster turns out to be a windfall.

In many ways, I am glad that Connie received some of the farm's money. It turned out that she was the only one to benefit from the farm's sixty-year history of blood, sweat, and tears. All the rest would go to future creditors. One should never rely on an inheritance to insure future prosperity. You just never know what can happen.

Jeff then began a series of misadventures. He sought a replacement for the female adoration with which he was accustomed since birth. He found a beautiful woman in Brazil who was fluent in three languages—Portuguese, Spanish, and English. I initially was against this move; however, she later proved through her efforts to help Jeff even after their divorce that she had a good spirit. I regret ever doubting her sincerity.

Our mother died in 2006 at the age of 87. The one person who was able to put some sensible limits on my brother's often freakishly grandiose plans passed away. Jeff was now not only going to race his steed—he was going to let that uncontrolled stallion run with wild abandon until it took flight in a flurry of manic decisions. He just never looked at the possible downside of his decisions.

Jeff had the estate, "the farm," given to him in its entirety by constructing a trust in which he was the sole beneficiary, to which my mother acquiesced. I did not ask about the will until about a month after my mother died. Jeff responded, "Well, Steve, that was all put in a trust long ago." He spoke in what I will call his feigned reasonable voice, like it was only reasonable that he would receive everything, while the rest of the family received zip.

I was miffed. I recognized that Jeff should have received the largest share, perhaps half of the estate. The other half should have been split up among the remaining five siblings. If this had taken place, in effect he would have received half the estate, while each of the remaining children would receive a tenth of the estate. He was not even going to give a token portion of the will to other members of the family. My father would never have done this.

We hear how a trust is so much better than probate. It would have been much better if the farm was apportioned according to law through probate. There is a wisdom to probate that should not be so easily dismissed.

Jeff received 100% of the inheritance and felt no doubt about the justice of that outcome. He did not even give a token to the rest of the family. It was a total slap in the face. The family wrote Jeff off.

I still maintained a dialogue with him, which would turn out to be a mistake. Valois and Lolly both indicated that I should have nothing to do with him. I did not listen and would later regret it. The moral of the story is to never contradict what two angels tell you to do. I gave Jeff way too much credit as being a basically decent human being.

Now that Jeff had replaced the first wife, he yearned to return to the high-flying gambling days. He could not stay away. I knew he would not be able to stay away because I knew from his childhood that he could not walk away from a losing situation. He had no one to drag him away from the contrived gambling game to keep him from losing all our money—at least he had no one he would listen to.

I just shook my head and resigned myself to the situation because it felt like fate was taking control. This situation was going to play out like a Greek tragedy. I felt dismissed that he did not ask me for some input. After all, I was the only one in the family still talking to him.

My mother died in 2006. By early 2008, Jeff was going to exercise the control and power over all the finances that was wrongfully denied to him, in his view, while my mother was alive. His inability to walk away from a bad deal would birth a catastrophe.

He bought a dive well away from the thriving metropolis of 15,000 people of Watertown, South Dakota. It never grew or contracted. I always felt uncomfortable with the place. I wanted to do all I could to avoid the restrictive, Watertown view of the world.

The future gambling place he bought was a bar on Lake Pelican. It was mostly a duck hunter's lake unlike the recreational and more popular Lake Kampeska, which was more accessible. The previous

Foxy's Casino was in the center of the mini-metropolis that Watertown was in South Dakota. The bar he bought at Pelican Lake was literally in the middle of nowhere. It was not even in a town in the middle of nowhere.

And then came the end of 2008 and the Great Recession. The biggest financial collapse since the Great Depression. Jeff's casino quickly went bankrupt. At one point, he decided to move the almost brand-new house he had built on the farm with his previous wife to the duck hunter's lake so he could carefully watch his employees stealing him blind. He ran out of money before relocating the house near his new and ill-fated casino. All he had left was an empty foundation on the farm and a broken-down new house on a lake next to his money-pit casino in the middle of nowhere.

Let's look at where I was after all of this, at the beginning of psychotherapy.

Chapter 23

The Antithesis

I went through a period of therapy when I came to a more jaundiced view of my family, which I refer to as the antithesis. The family appeared the following way in my antithesis view:

1. My father was a hard-working man that my mother stressed to the limit so that his genetic predisposition to bipolar disorder was revealed. My mother was mainly to blame. I think I was being overly harsh on my mother because I felt she was overly harsh on my father. I used to beg her to stop the fighting, realizing that she was the only one cognizant enough to be able to exert some form of self-control.

2. My mother hid behind the farm because of insecurity. She bore a large family of eight to have a workforce on the farm at her disposal. There were other reasons to be sure, and she loved us in her way, but I was not at the point in therapy where I could clearly see that.

3. My eldest sister, Valois, was an angel from heaven. This is probably the one unchanging fact in the family. *The Course in Miracles* teaches that whatever is real is eternal and immutable. So be it.

4. My third oldest sister, Kathy, had a genetic predisposition to depressive psychosis. She saw the world through the lens of the farm. In farm logic, you put up with difficult circumstances, like an alcoholic husband, because that was the way life was. I think the farm prepared us all to put up with more abuse than a

person should. It was hard for us to see abuse in situations that were demonstrably better than the social-emotional pit we were raised in as a child.

5. I thought of my eldest brother, Alan, as simply the Beast. He was a sadistic animal who beat and humiliated me because he enjoyed it. He seemed larger than life because he was three times larger and ten times stronger than I was. I failed to see what a weak coward a bully is. They only pick on those who muster no resistance to them. I could have tried to counter-terrorize him (hit him over the head with a frying pan?), but I believed at the time that he would have escalated his torture of me in response.

6. My second oldest brother, Greg, was a lost soul who was never taught how to live. He swallowed the farm's materialistic values hook, line, and sinker. I actually liked Greg, and he would become a different person when he was away from Alan. There was so little regard to the children having lives separate from the farm. If the work was done, that was all I felt mattered to my mother.

7. My fourth oldest sister, Lolly, received no guidance or affection from our parents. She was prone to seek the affection she never received from her parents from a boyfriend. After a short and disastrous first marriage in which she had a baby girl, she married her current husband. They have been married for thirty years and have five children. The farm affected her, but, somehow, she managed to hit the reset button on her attitudes.

8. Despite my mother's insistence that I was a dead ringer for my maternal grandfather, I had no similarity to him. I was an abstract thinker who somehow was thrown into the materialistic survival game of the farm. I resolved to study and become the most abstract-thinking professional I could conjure, a clinical psychologist, living entirely in my head and in

the heads of others. Given my family, I do not think the choice of a mental health profession was random. It is interesting that my mother insisted that we have little to do with my father's family who were university professors, civil engineers, priests, etc. She wanted us to spend all our extended family time with her close relatives, who had no professionals and too many alcoholics.

9. My youngest brother, Jeff, was worshipped by my mom. The thinking was like the Divine Child archetype that often appears in dreams. In this archetype, the Divine Child, Jeff, had all the hopes and desires of my mother projected onto him. He became the Messiah figure who would "save the farm." We did not realize that he was like a black hole from which no light would emerge. The only thing infant-like or babyish about him was his total narcissism and lack of regard for others. The only thing magical about him was his ability to make the farm's assets disappear. It would take a while for me, with the help of therapy, to finally see what kind of person I was actually dealing with. The only thing divine about him was, how in God's name did he do it (bring so much destruction to everyone)?

Developing understanding and forgiveness of my family members was helped through dream interpretation, which became a significant part of my psychotherapy and path to healing.

Chapter 24

Dream On

My therapist, Darlene, was excellent. She was a social worker who was trained at the Dr. Carl Jung Institute in Zurich, Switzerland. Carl Jung started this training facility for dream interpretation according to his theory. I believe Jung's theory of personality best describes what occurs in dreams.

Jung was originally a follower of Freud. Sigmund Freud was fixated on sex and aggression as being the primary instincts. Jung had a more expanded view that included altruism, spirituality, and the idea that we are all connected in some way, which he called the collective unconscious. We, of course, have our individual subconscious, each of which feeds into the collective unconscious. The best way to peer into the subconscious is to look closely at our dreams, which is when social censorship is lifted.

When we are asleep, the subconscious in symbolic form presents what is really going on, which we have not seen before because we repress thoughts that are unpleasant. The idea of a collective unconscious is fascinating; it implies that not all the images in dreams are ours alone. Some images may be visitors from the collective unconscious (collective subconscious).

We do not know how this happens other than to say that it seems that all human minds are connected. I believe that someday science will discover how this connectedness occurs. I am open to the idea that it may happen on the level of another dimension; there are eight dimensions we have not experienced, according to theoretical physicists.

Jungian therapists can be wizards at dream interpretation if they are skilled. The German Jungian dream interpretation analyst, Marie-Louise von Franz, one of the great original Jungian therapists, thought that dream interpretation was the only way we could directly look at the individual person's subconscious. I could not agree more. Trying to determine what is happening in a person's subconscious from what they are saying consciously is once removed and fraught with error.

My fascination with dreams has grown to the point that I am almost bored with behavioral and cognitive therapy approaches. Do not misunderstand me. I believe those therapies have much to offer. They work best when one already knows what the problem is.

Sometimes, what should be done consciously to solve a problem is plain to see. It follows conscious deductive logic. I used to be a math major at one point as an undergraduate, was a statistics minor in graduate school, and received computer training in the past. Conscious logic and rational thinking were never a problem for me.

Fascination with subconscious irrational thinking has been the Holy Grail for me. Once one reaches the point where subconscious influences are vetted, usually 70% to 80% of therapy goals are accomplished. Typically, cognitive and behavioral therapies work best once ways are found to get beyond the client's subconscious, self-defeating resistances. Seeing that psychodynamic therapies bring us closer to the heart of conflicts, I have continued to drift into abstract subconscious approaches involving dream work.

As a result of interest in psychodynamic therapies and my own personal therapy, which was primarily dream interpretation, my thinking about how to interpret dreams became more clear. I had always been at least adequate at interpreting dreams, but did not really feel good about it until I had been practicing it for ten years. After I had been interpreting dreams for twenty years, I felt that I was offering interpretations that were truly enlightening.

Clients that knew me for years began to bring in dreams, telling me, "This is how you are going to interpret this dream." When I asked how they knew what I would say, they would virtually always say some version of, "Because that is what you always say with this type of dream." I realized that I was using a set of rules to interpret dreams.

Dreams are very complex and have many levels. The way I interpret dreams is at what I call the first level of dream interpretation. That is where I assume each living thing or spirit in a person's dream represents a part of the person's mind. I have found that dreams use gender as a code, with males going more with an action part of the mind, and females going more with an emotion part of the psyche. In my experience, this holds true whether you are heterosexual, lesbian, gay, transsexual, bisexual, or otherwise.

What I describe in the previous paragraph are the first two rules in my book, *Dreams: Guide to the Soul.* (The book is available at http://www.drstevenfox.com.) There are forty rules in all. Three or four dream examples are given to illustrate each rule. The book uses Jungian dream interpretation extensively. One of Carl Jung's most helpful ideas was the concept of archetypes.

An archetype is a pattern of thought that has been handed down through the generations by the connectedness of human consciousness. It is a radical idea—any thought that any human has ever had over the course of millennia could be in the collective unconscious. This includes such archetypes as father, mother, heroic masculine, queen, savage masculine, trickster, shadow, the divine child, the willing sacrifice, and so forth. It is a shorthand method of identifying complex repetitive patterns of thoughts and actions within dreams. It adds a richness and complexity that straight Freudian dream interpretations cannot match.

My dream interpretation blog is at http://www.drfoxblog.com. I am one of four or so main dream interpreters on "The Power of Dreams" board started by Dale Miesen on Facebook, where we have about 10,000 followers. There is almost nothing I would rather do than interpret dreams.

I am experienced at interpreting dreams, being a private practice psychologist with over thirty years of experience (if you count my graduate school experience during which I saw clients—it would be over 35 years of experience). As I write this, I am surprised that I do not feel older than I do, especially given that I have multiple sclerosis. Meeting with clients, trying to change their life and sometimes their soul, is an experience in witnessing people face their darkest fears. Unexpectedly, I personally feel rejuvenated participating with sincere clients in this life-affirming endeavor.

All my life, I wanted to be known for being able to interpret dreams. It is easily the most interesting work I participate in. After twenty years of practice, my thoughts about dreams coalesced in such a way that I believe clients usually received interpretations that went well beyond the obvious because of my experience in doing dream interpretation psychotherapy. The result of this experience was my book *Dreams: Guide to the Soul,* which was published in 2013.

Dreams: Guide to the Soul describes my system of interpreting dreams. As explained earlier, I use forty guidelines or rules, and the book was based on anonymous client dreams in which details were changed to protect the innocent. I included two of my own dreams in which details were changed to protect two male members of my family. After recent events, I will no longer try to protect them and present events as they actually happened.

The description of the human-angel dream that gave me four rules to live by to send the MS into remission was described previously in this book. Another such dream, described in *Dreams: Guide to the Soul,* signaled when I was ready to run during my initial recovery from the

MS. The other two dreams involved my oldest brother Alan and my younger brother Jeff. I had thought of Alan as the abusive Beast in the past. I had thought of Jeff as the Divine Child in the past, which is one of the Jungian archetypes. This was a misnomer. Jeff was actually closer to the Trickster archetype.

It is interesting how I now think of Alan as a confused and misdirected savage masculine energy. Presently, and even more surprising to me, is that I now see Jeff as a wheeler-dealer con-man. Alan benefits from my overall analysis of family dynamics, and specifically in how I have examined our family of origin affecting him. Conversely, Jeff is seen more negatively, though more clearly, because of recent events. These recent events confirm that I was blinded by my loyalty to this brother with whom I was left surviving on the farm after my two older brothers were forced to leave when their beatings went too far. Insight continues throughout our lifetime, and the clarity of these insights becomes grander as we age.

The Alan Dream: Giving the Savage Masculine What-For

When I was around 37, I dreamt that I was in my hometown Catholic church. My family and my then-abusive brother Alan had their backs to me. Alan handed me a note denying any abuse ever occurred.

I knew that Alan's view of events was in complete agreement with my mother's opinion. I responded with a note that I personally handed Alan, detailing the truth of the abuse as I saw it. A chorus of animas (models of the ideal woman), three attractive women at the front of the church, then sang the "Truth" to Alan in a jazzy, rabble-rousing, *Chicago* style. One anima with brown and loosely curled, Rembrandt-style hair was really into it. She sang in Alan's face as loudly and insultingly as she possibly could.

My Interpretation: Reclaiming My Energy

I made a breakthrough when I wrote letters that I sent to the abuser, Alan, that described the situation as I lived it. I told him that I forgave him because I wanted to reclaim the energy for my life that I had previously wasted on hating him. The main reason I forgave him was for my benefit.

I needed to reclaim that wasted energy. I also came to realize that there was a shadow part of myself that was hugely angry over the abuse. By forgiving Alan for my sake, I was able to quiet the anger and use that energy for positive purposes, such as healing myself and writing this book.

The three beautiful sisters were the three sane sisters I had to cushion the effects of the abuse. Particularly in the cases of Valois (twelve years older than me) and Lauretta (one year older than me); I credit them for keeping me mostly mentally healthy. The animas in the dream were archetypal or ideal women who appeared very classic, while also looking like a combination of Valois and Lauretta (Lolly) in appearance.

The Jeff Dream: The Wheeler-Dealer Loses It All

I had this dream in 1998, five years after my father's death (Alois Fox, 8/16/1915—5/21/1993) at the age of 77. It was eight years prior to my mother's (Lauretta Fox, 8/4/1918—4/13/2006) death at the age of 87. It was a predictive dream of what would ultimately happen with my brother Jeff and the farm.

I dreamed Jeff, who was four years younger than me, was trimming the hooves of a prize-winning Holstein show-cow named Snowy while I watched from a short distance. Jeff was trimming the cow's hooves in a very unusual way. The cow was thrown down on a large piece of plywood across an old and worn-out carpenter's bench in a clumsy and almost impossibly difficult setup.

Suddenly our two older brothers, Alan and Greg, who looked like professional wrestlers, appeared, and ran toward me, the dreamer. The animal was startled and jumped up in a commotion. Jeff moved to the side and was unhurt. My father was in the background and tried to warn me to get out of there as fast as I could.

I was mesmerized by the situation and felt like I could not move. The cow then staggered like an intoxicated alcoholic toward me. I was very worried that the cow might stumble and fall on me.

My Interpretation: Give Up on the Relationship with Jeff Before It Is Too Late

The hardest thing to remember in dream work is that at the first and intrapsychic level of interpretation, each character and animal in the dream represents a part of the dreamer's psyche. I had worked hard on my father's farm in my youth, and throughout college and graduate school. I subsequently went to live in Albany, New York, and worked as a clinical psychologist.

My brother Jeff stayed on the farm and rented the land out while pursuing additional businesses, such as carpet cleaning, a restaurant, and ultimately a casino, which came to consume almost all his time and energy. Jeff used the farm and its possessions as equity, which allowed him to buy and build the various businesses. He also did some investing in rental properties for my mother.

He decided, in his Divine Child reasoning, that he alone would inherit 100% of the property by putting the farm in a trust with himself as the executor. He later felt charitable for letting Alan's daughter raid Mom's ramshackle mobile home on the farm for some trinkets and jewelry. He felt quite righteous about letting some junk go. What a disgrace.

Jeff was totally unleashed after our parents died. He made a series of increasingly risky investments and refused to walk away from any bad deal. He went through the entire inheritance in about a year. His ultimate undoing was the casinos he bought. Then came the Great Recession of 2008 which put the final nail in the coffin of his business endeavors. He was thoroughly drained of money.

Looking at the dream psychologically, Jeff represented the part of me that dealt with Jeff and the farm in my adult years. Trimming the cow's hooves meant my ego was trying to get me to trim my instinctive support of the farm (the cow supports the farm financially). The hooves support the cow (my instincts), which is vital to the farm materially and physically. The whole gist of the dream is that I was instinctively hell-bent to support the farm in whatever way I could. The cows were the money producers for the farm, and trimming the hooves was advice from the dream to cut back on my instinctive support of the farm.

The dream was warning me: trying to help the farm or Jeff financially was misguided. My instinctive desire to help my brother and mother was not going to work. I had obsessively and needlessly worried about mom and Jeff's financial health. The farm was a trap that could hurt me because it mesmerized me. It, and my attachments to Jeff and my mother, had an unhealthy hold on me at that stage in my life.

My two older, physically abusive brothers were huge and menacing in the dream. Their sudden appearance startled the cow, which was saying the shadow abusers deeply scared me too, to the point that my instincts (the cow) became unsteady. I had remnant anxiety from the physical abuse I suffered as a child until I was in my fifties.

The whole setup (the workbench and plywood) was emblematic of the farm's structure both cognitively and emotionally. No good was to come from it. My instinct to help my family and the farm was likely to result in my getting hurt from Jeff "trimming," that is, skimming the farm financially.

The dream predicted that I was likely to get hurt by the situation. That the cow staggered like a drunken alcoholic was a warning that my instincts did not see the situation clearly and that I was addicted to the farm and what it represented to me. The farm held serious problems ever since I can remember.

It is notable that my father was a disabled man who was mostly ignored by abusers, with some infrequent exceptions, and terrorized by his wife. There was no love left in the marriage by the time I was a teenager. The children were raised like a cash crop to work on the farm and keep it going.

The cow's name, Snowy, was significant, as every detail in a dream can be important and virtually is never random. In dreams, water is almost always emotion. Snow is frozen water, therefore, cold emotion. The cow being named Snowy is another case of the dream making even little details close to perfect. The emotion on the farm was mostly cold.

My father did have a relationship with me. My father was the one who finally called the sheriff after the abusers went overboard and inflicted painful physical blows. The abuse stopped after the intervention by the courts. My father had his faults and was untreated bipolar, but he was an essentially decent man who saved me.

Back in 1998, with the help of therapy, I was able to avoid being tricked into giving Jeff more of my money prior to my mother's death. Unbelievably, Jeff and mom constantly bewailed their supposedly poor financial condition to me. By listening to the message of my dream, I resisted my ingrained dysfunctional instinct to help them by giving my energy away to them when they did not need it. Jeff was a liar who self-righteously proclaimed that he and he alone was the only one deserving of an inheritance. True to form, after the bankruptcy, Jeff continued to ask me and relatives for money to support his ventures. He was looking for a substitute for his bankrupt gravy train, the farm. As will be seen further in the next chapter, we should always pay close attention to dreams.

Chapter 25

Things Deteriorate to Horrible with Aftermath:

I Learn to Stop Disbelieving My Dreams

Jeff sold all the valuable farmland to the City of Watertown for about a half million dollars so that he could throw it all into the second hopeless casino. The farmland was located near a major interchange of Interstate 29 and Highway 212. The land continued to appreciate since it was sold to the city. It turned out that the smartest thing to do with the land would have been simply to rent it out to farmers. By 2015, farmland almost everywhere had almost doubled in price.

Jeff's bankruptcy and refusal to deal with the situation realistically led to his second wife divorcing him. He truly loved her. He eventually obtained a job selling potato chips and snacks to grocery stores for a major corporation.

He said his employer made him buy a new car for the position. He said he was transferred to Florida and then he was fired only weeks after he moved so that a more senior employee could take his position. As subsequent events will show, there are many reasons to doubt his self-reports.

Jeff was now skilled in helping things go from worse to horrible. He started selling furniture at a store, but could not make enough money to live on since he was paid mainly on commission. He actually had to go to a food pantry to get some food to eat. He was not able to sell things in a catastrophic economy.

He lived in a trailer. His ex-wife moved to Florida and rented a mobile home several blocks from him. She helped him out as much as she could. Jeff, of course, continued to use her as much as he could.

I questioned her sincerity before they were married. After she contacted me several times because she was worried about Jeff's situation, I stopped questioning her motives. I felt empathy for both of them as they were reeling in the consequences of Jeff's hasty decisions.

The bankruptcy continued to follow Jeff. The court allowed him to keep six thousand dollars of possessions on condition that he pay off the six thousand over time. Jeff did not have enough to live on, let alone pay back six thousand, or so I was told.

He asked me to help him. I gave him enough to fend off the payments until he could get situated. I felt like I slipped back into my role of trying to save the farm. If I would have continued in therapy, I do not think I would have made that mistake. It is important to not quit therapy prematurely. Change can occur without therapy with effort sometimes, but it will probably take longer.

At that time, unbelievably, I still felt loyal to Jeff. If I become loyal to a person, that loyalty dies hard. On the farm, we were a team who made the farm survive after the departure of my two older brothers. I engaged in many telephone discussions with him in 2014 trying to figure out how he could dig himself out of the hole he had created.

In 2015, Jeff contacted me several times in desperation. I ended up giving him money, so he could be trained as a trucker and cover some bills. He did get the training as a trucker, but actually used a substantial portion of the money I gave him to try to get some woman to move to the United States so that he could get into her newly acquired inheritance. The woman turned out to be a scam. The original scammer, Jeff, was out-scammed. He had learned nothing. I learned never to trust him again. I should have listened to my two angel sisters.

Jeff lived his life as a fantasy set up for him by the work of others. First, his fantasy was built on the work of those in the family. Our mother gave him the farm as insurance for having a caretaker in her old age. He returned to financial reality with a thump.

I felt his unbelievable journey was now ending with a takeover of harsh reality. I felt significantly less resentment after seeing how this Shakespearean tragedy played out. Justice was eventually served. The money he received from the farm turned out to be a Trojan horse that took down his fantasy empire from within. I had to face the reality I had wanted to deny for so long—he was now nothing more than a ruthless conman.

From 2010 to 2014, I did not hear much from Jeff, and was glad I did not hear from him. In 2015, he contacted me out of desperation. He had leftover bills he still had to pay from the bankruptcy court. He had been through a series of jobs and was living near his ex from Brazil in Florida. She still came in handy as a person to use. I felt kinship with her.

At my urging, he went to truck driving school and obtained a commercial license so that he could drive semi-trucks. I loaned him money to satisfy the courts, get a place to live, and pay for his truck driver training. I even helped him get reasonable health insurance through Obamacare. Altogether, I loaned him about $8,000.

After the final loan, he never again communicated with me by phone, mail, email, or text as we had done before. He never paid back one cent of the $8,000 I loaned him. I was finally done with him.

The mistake I made was that by 2015, I thought he had changed. More accurately, I wanted to believe that he had changed. Looking back at the dream I had in 1998, the dream accurately predicted seven years earlier what would happen if I continued to believe in his projects. Old habits die hard. I resolved to really follow my dreams from this point forward. The inner voice of my subconscious never leads me astray, though it's sometimes difficult to trust or listen when the message is not what I hope to hear.

I want to take you forward by showing you the archangels I use to make positive accomplishments.

Chapter 26

Choosing Your Angels

I personally have found that including angels, positive spirits, and saints in prayer increases the effect of prayer. Each person has a vast array of angels to choose from for assistance. The angels only have one requirement for enlisting their help—you must ask the angel to help. That's it.

It is simple enough, but people resist asking for help. It takes humility to recognize how difficult life is, and how we sometimes, or often, need help. You must overcome the narcissistic feeling internalized from society that upholds the ridiculous ideal that you alone can solve all your problems. There is no shame in asking the spiritual realm for help. It is in fact a divine gift that spiritual forces are willing and able to help us.

Which angels do you ask to help? It depends on who you are and what you need. I want to give you the angels I use and the reasons for asking these specific angels to help me. I believe this knowledge helps us discern which angel to appeal to in our prayers. In that way, we can marshal the forces to help us.

The special angels I found to be most helpful were as follows:

1. **Azrael** is the angel of death. In dreams, each character is a different part of the dreamer's mind at the first level of dream interpretation. When a character in one's dream dies, it is usually a signal that part of your mind/character/personality needs to die. This "death" usually is a message from the subconscious that the part of the persona represented by the

dying character needs to be deemphasized so that other parts of the personality can become more prominent. I needed Azrael because I needed to let past parts of myself die, especially the angry and embittered parts of my personality, due to the abuse. The venom that deep resentments produce within a person can emotionally, and eventually physically, kill us. We must let those angry, frustrated parts die so the positive and loving parts of our mind command our actions. Forgiveness is not an altruistic gesture—it is an action necessary to set free the bombs and mines we have set in our own minds that will cause an illness to detonate when we are under stress. Azrael was needed for the discernment necessary to determine which personality parts needed to die.

2. **Jophiel** is the angel of beauty. Specifically, her focus is on showing beauty of thoughts, intentions, and attitudes. She is the exemplar of healing rule number two imparted to my wife by an angel in a dream. The rule was to ***Show Inner Beauty*** as an important part of my healing. Jophiel was needed for the discernment necessary to determine which personality parts needed to be born, emphasized, and prioritized. The other important part was not to be embarrassed or reticent about showing positive qualities and having self-esteem about them.

3. **Metatron** is a very special angel who is thought of as the Angel of Life because he once was human. He was the grandfather of Noah, named Enoch. He is special to children because he led the children out of Israel and stopped Abraham from sacrificing his son, Isaac. He is special to writers in my mind because he was the "recording angel" or "celestial scribe," who kept the Akashic records, an archive on which all human history of thoughts and deeds are written. I think of him as guarding my inner child, as being especially aware of the hardships of life for humans, and as being the ultimate

writer who records the truth of all happenings. I invoked Metatron's intercession when writing this book.

4. **Raziel** is the angel of divine wisdom. He can reveal these holy secrets with God's permission—this allows him to aid supplicants. He helps people access divine wisdom to gain deeper insight to solve their problems. Helping mankind understand the secrets of the universe with divinely guided intuition to solve problems is his specialty. I think of him as helping me to use empathy correctly and unconditionally.

5. **Ariel** is the angel of nature. She protects the earth's animals, plants, and elements (fire, water, and wind). She helps God's creatures (both wild and domestic) and the environment heal. She works with Raphael (one of the Big Three archangels discussed previously) when healing is involved. I think of my love of nature, plants, and pets (especially when pets are ill) when I think of Ariel. I think of Rafael as providing more direct healing, while Ariel ensures that our environment (which includes plants, animals, and the elements of wind, water, and fire) will be maximally conducive to healing. Ariel is a very earthy angel that improves the conditions of nature so that healing is more likely to occur.

6. **Jeremiel** is the angel that helps us to understand our dreams. He is also involved in life review—looking at our personal past and learning from the lessons life has taught us through experience. He is an angel who helps guide dream interpretation. I believe he was an important part of my writing an extensive book on dream interpretation, which I believe introduces a host of important vital innovative ideas in dream work. The book, of course, is *Dreams: Guide to the Soul* (http://www.drstevenfox.com).

I urge you to connect with the Big Three archangels (Michael, Raphael, and Gabriel) plus the other archangels (or major angels) that fit your personality and specific situation. There are also your everyday working angels, who are there to help whenever you seek assistance in a certain area in your life. They have been assigned to you, and will intervene when you ask for help, but you do not have to ask for them by their formal name because they are always with you, every day.

Chapter 27

Everyday Angels

Everyday angels are unlike the major angels or archangels who must be asked by name for help. To use a metaphor, your everyday angels are like members of your family who are ready and nearby to help you (who frequently are there to help you whether you have asked them or not); whereas, archangels or major angels are like a Senator or Congressman who can help you but must be asked in a more formal way. They are, for the time, simply closer to the President (God) than you are.

Everyone has a staff of angels, like a family of angels, that serve everyday needs. The most well-known is your **guardian angel**. Your guardian angel is your personal protector and your go-to angel for a myriad of purposes.

Your **personal healing angel** is the most important angel in overcoming chronic disease. Decisions regarding your health are the concern of your personal healing angel. Choices to improve your health such as diet, exercise, or alternative treatments are best made with this angel as a consultant. Especially important are choices regarding medical treatments you can either reject or pursue.

Your **helper angel** is an all-around utility fielder. He or she is focused on whatever goals need help in your life. He is an all-around booster who works in conjunction with your other personal angels.

Your **teacher angel** is mainly important when teaching new information to learners. I think of this angel as vital when it is necessary for me to be empathic with the difficulty of teaching lessons to others. Such work makes me regret my elementary smart-mouthed rebellion when teachers tried to teach me important material as a child.

The **joy angel** is especially important after tragedies. She/he reminds us that there is an essential joy to life that must be appreciated and re-appreciated. This angel can help keep us from viewing life as dreary and endless torture.

I think of the **master guide** as the personal guidance master who gives fatherly advice. He usually is a master of the ways of the world. He typically focuses more on actions we can take to repair a situation or rehabilitate ourselves. In desperate situations that require immediate action, the master guide gives reliable direction.

One of the most useful angels is the **runner angel**. He/she literally hits the ground running. This is the angel to call when we need to avoid little hassles. Finding parking spaces, getting tickets to an event or concert, getting accepted to a program you have applied to, locating a missing object, checking in for plane flights, etc., are the kinds of issues this angel deals with. The runner angel will work hard to smooth your journeys.

Angels are one kind of spiritual helper that I have learned to connect with in my healing journey. Another kind of spiritual helper consists of saints and religious icons. I consider the next chapter on saints and icons to be my favorite. It involves saintly figures of different religions and persuasions.

Chapter 28

Saints and Icons

There is a plethora of saints from which to enlist spiritual assistance and intercession. These saints are not worshipped, but are co-supplicants in helping the person with multiple sclerosis ask for help. The saints used depend upon your needs. You want to choose saints that are experts in an area in which you particularly need help. The icons are that and much more, and will be discussed toward the end of this chapter. What follows is my short list of saints whom I have asked for assistance in intercession with God:

1. **Saint Francis** in my mind is the saint of animals, birds, the environment, and helping the poor and indigent. He was born wealthy and even was in the military before starting his monkhood. He was known for giving whatever he had to the poor. Birds and animals were tranquil and at peace around St. Francis of Assisi, which is a town in Italy. He lived around 1200 A.D. and died in his early forties. Pope Francis has taken his namesake to heart, and his main message has been for the Catholic Church to be less regal and more concerned with the plight of the poor, the marginalized, and the immigrants, particularly in the wealthy country of the United States. There is enough wealth in the USA that no one should be homeless or hungry. Pope Francis, true to his namesake, gave a speech to a joint session of the United States Congress urging legislators to do more to reduce climate change because of the devastating effects it is having upon the earth. Pope Francis was the first pope I saw dine with the homeless instead of with members of

Congress. There is a message in his decision to eat with the poor that no one missed.

2. **Saint Teresa of Avila** for me is a saint of miracles that can be accomplished when we put our mind to it. She is also seen by me as an exemplar of the virtues of long-suffering patience in the face of illness. She lived in the 1500s and died when she was about 67 years old. She was a mystic who greatly expanded the Catholic Church's concept of what can be accomplished spiritually through prayer. She described methods of prayer that ultimately lead to states of ecstasy. During these ultimate states of ecstasy, she lightened her body to the point that she would levitate. It was said that she would sometimes levitate during the Catholic mass. There were reports that the nuns in her cloister sometimes had to hold her down to stop the levitation. She was sick much of her life, but saw her illness as a gift from God. She famously said, "Let me suffer or let me die." She considered such suffering to be for the glory of God. She was a mystic's mystic.

3. **Saint Germaine** is a New Age saint who is considered one of the ascended masters. He lived from 1710 until 1784. The legend behind this ascended master is that he was Sir Francis Bacon who faked his death, located in Transylvania, and acquired magical powers. I came across him from my acquaintance with a New Age massage therapist who instructed myself, my wife, and a group of perhaps six psychologists in using visualization of different colors of light. The two lights that relieved my symptoms the most were green light from Archangel Rafael and the violet flame of Saint Germaine. I accept healing from any source as long as the thoughts and intentions are mostly going up and not going down.

4. **Padre Pio** was born in Italy and came from a humble background. He lived to be 81 years old, from 1887 until 1968. Because of the extreme and supernatural miracles attributed to

him, the Church did not canonize him until forty-four years after his death. He was said to give vision to a girl who had no pupils. Other monks testified that he had the ability of bilocation. During World War II, many Air Force pilots turned back from bombing San Giovanni Rotondo in Italy because they said they saw a monk appear in the sky telling them to go back. He was finally canonized in 2002. He is a favorite saint of mine because he did the impossible. I was told, over and over, that there was no cure for multiple sclerosis and that I would end up in a wheelchair. The Catholic Church, with its canonization of Padre Pio, agreed in their theology that anything is possible. To get over a chronic illness like MS, one must believe the impossible is possible.

5. **Jesus Christ** is an icon, of course, who must be included in my list. His many healing miracles are a constant inspiration. When he spoke of his miracles, he made sure to spread the message that all of these (miracles) and more can be accomplished by any of us through faith.

6. **Buddha** is on my list for his iconic and inspiring views on ending suffering through meditation and by stopping the seemingly endless, mindless monkey-chatter that occupies our minds. Ending the cycle of suffering by realizing the nature of life and resolving to take what action we can to be happy is ultimately sensible. Moderation encouraged by Buddhists might have saved my brothers.

Chapter 29

The Synthesis

After therapy, and seeing and reflecting upon the events that occurred throughout my life, I have come to a synthesis. The synthesis is as follows:

1. My father had bipolar disorder all my life, it just became more severe as the years progressed. He finally was diagnosed in his sixties. There was such a dearth of mental health services in South Dakota that being treated for mental health meant you were in the state hospital in Yankton, South Dakota. Neither my father nor my mother had a clue about what was happening. He was basically a good German from an educated family that included a priest, an engineer, a civil servant, and a noted professor. His life was torn up by a mostly genetic disorder—he could not deal well with stress. I felt like he was a wounded lion who was powerful too early in his life. His father died when he was thirteen. He was the oldest boy on a farm with six kids and his mother. He worked on the farm during the day and in a meat-packing plant at night during the Depression. The bipolar disorder was probably adaptive at that point in his life before it became severe later. I wish I would have realized what was going on with him sooner. I guess I was under the spell of the family myth. These rampant mental health problems in my family explain why I became so interested in psychology and subconscious processes.

2. My mother was an asocial being who probably was a person with high-functioning Asperger's disorder. Social autism marks

this disorder. It is notable that she had a sister, Darlene, who spent most of her life living with her parents. Darlene sat in one place, did not talk, and was fascinated with tearing small pieces of paper from magazines and twirling them for hours. My maternal grandparents told people she "fell out of the crib as a baby." The truth was that Darlene was autistic on the day she was born. My grandparents just never met with a mental health professional who could have imparted the autism diagnosis to them. My mother was a good woman who could never figure out why life handed her the problems she experienced. It is amazing that she was able to withstand all the stress that she did. I feel she had much to offer the world and did the best she could. A hurricane of children and mental illness confounded her. The most valuable thing I learned from my mother was to keep putting one foot in front of the other—no matter what. When down and out, perseverance and a long-suffering attitude will carry the day, or most importantly, carry life forward.

3. My eldest sister, Valois, was an angel from heaven. I want to give you an update on Valois. She was a beautiful woman who became a registered nurse. She married a doctor, an anesthesiologist, who later became wealthy and bought a hospital with partners. They had eight children who were very successful. Her children and grandchildren thank God almost daily on Facebook that Valois is their mother/grandmother. As my once-eighth-grade, eighty-year-old English teacher said after asking me if Valois was my sister, "My mind just lights up when I think of Valois."

4. My third oldest sister, Kathy, had the farm view of life that did not prepare her for the stressors she endured, which included an alcoholic husband. Kathy decompensated into psychosis. I felt the loss of a sister who never fully realized how much trouble she was in. I think there had to be a big genetic

component involved with her decompensation, although I feel that the family stress negatively affected her psychodynamics.

5. My eldest brother, Alan, was not really a beast. He was the oldest boy who was most severely affected by my father's downfall. Alan remembered a time when our father functioned relatively well. He acted beastly toward the brother that most resembled his father and the extended paternal family in looks and brains—me. I hated him for a long time, but I no longer hate him. I mostly feel sorry for him, for our family, and I guess for myself. Life is so overwhelmingly hard at times, harder than I would have ever believed when I was young.

6. Greg reacted to the war between my parents by acting out, shoplifting, running long distances, and ditching school. He tragically died in his early fifties when the semi-truck he drove lost brakes and plunged over a steep cliff in the Rocky Mountains. I felt his demise was the ultimate loss of a lost soul. He never was able to take another worldview inside himself. He was left acting out conflicts that have no resolution unless you go within. His life was a strong argument for going to therapy or doing something to go within and resolve inner conflicts.

7. My sister, Lolly, was a social woman everyone loved. She found the love she needed outside of the home. After she divorced the man who helped her escape from the farm, she married the love of her life, became a registered nurse, and had six children. She found religion and spirituality, which helped her direct her energy positively. I always felt that Lolly and Valois were the two angels who stopped my descent towards hell. It was their empathy, compassion, and understanding that makes me strongly biased favorably toward women.

8. It became clear to me what a wide divergence there was between my mother's extended family and my father's

extended family. My mother's family did not benefit from the comparison. It was plain to see, as was said in olden times, that my father married beneath him. This was more than a difference in socio-economic standing. The concept of the purpose of a family is central here. My father's side of the family believed in raising a child to prepare him for life as an adult, contributing to the larger world. My mother's side of the family implicitly saw children as subjects to be dealt with fully in the here and now, without regard to any vision the child may have of the future, of life outside of and beyond the family.

9. What happened to my younger brother, the eighth of eight children, was a Greek tragedy that the rest of the family could only feel was poetic justice. The fall of Jeff's empire was a lesson in karma. He found that what he made go around came back around, vigorously.

In the next chapters, I want to present a plethora of methods I used to improve my health. All of them contributed to improvement until I reached a tipping point. I think, especially with chronic disease, that the treatment methods need to reach a critical mass of positive effect, before the corner is turned on the disease and remission ensues. You won't know which methods work until you try them and see how your body reacts.

Chapter 30

Tai Chi and Becoming Aware of Body Language

Tai Chi is a martial art based on gentle, rhythmic, neuro-physical exercise. These rhythmic, slow motions are often performed daily by the Chinese in public near the street. There is almost nothing strenuous about the moves, so Tai Chi is ideal for the elderly and those with compromised health. I believe it is useful for neural integration, especially for movement disorders like multiple sclerosis and Parkinson's disease.

I once was at a workshop by noted Jungian (follower of Dr. Carl Jung) analyst Marion Woodman. She is an extremely gifted analyst, especially regarding feminine psychology. This is epitomized by one of her many excellent books, *The Ravaged Bridegroom*.

I attended one of her many workshops in my quest to become an expert in dream interpretation. At some point, she had members of the audience pair up. One person was to make movements, while the other person interpreted and encouraged the other's movements. I interpreted his movements mostly by using Tai Chi as a model. For example, I encouraged him to "pull the energy down" when he reached for the sky. He ended up making a circular motion with his hands raised and then moving his arms downward. It was somehow exciting and invigorating.

I also had another occasion to publicly evaluate and use body language. As I became more engrossed in dream work, I noticed that the more I interpreted dreams, the more intuitive I became. I began to seek out opportunities to exercise my intuition on a professional basis. At some point, I decided to attend a continuing education psychology seminar hosted by the Milton Erickson Institute in Phoenix, Arizona.

Milton Erickson was an intuitive and master hypnotist who was severely disabled due to polio. He spent much of his time sitting in a wheelchair and observing people's behavior. This observation informed many of his techniques. His approach focused largely on body language.

The presenter at the conference at the workshop I attended demonstrated an interesting technique. He asked a volunteer from the audience to stand on the stage, close his eyes, and remember the most traumatic incident in his life. When the volunteer reached the point where the trauma was fully remembered in all its detail, he was to raise a finger.

After the volunteer signaled that he had reached the height of his trauma by raising his finger, the presenter stared intently at the man's face. He then described in detail the emotions the presenter could discern the volunteer was feeling while the volunteer continued to think of the trauma with his eyes closed. When the presenter felt he could say nothing new, he asked the volunteer if what the presenter said was close to what the volunteer felt.

He replied, "That was not only close, that was exactly what I felt."

When he was done, the presenter asked for another interpreter from the audience to do the same thing with a new volunteer. Taking my heart into my hands, I offered to be the temporary translator of emotion I viewed in another. My volunteer was a young, attractive woman.

The descriptions I gave of her facial expressions were easy. She was very expressive emotionally. Her first facial expression was one of personal violation. I quickly decided she was reacting to either a mugging, a beating, or a rape.

It was a lesson to me that the feelings to each of these events probably have a similar emotional basis. At the heart of her facial expression was the feeling of being personally violated. She also had the look of being surprised. I suspected that someone violated her whom she had previously trusted, which could be a family member or something like a date rape.

When I was finished, I asked her if what I described was close to what she was feeling. She stated, "That was not only close, that was exactly what I was feeling." This was in the early 1990s when I hit my stride as a therapist. I was pleased that by going to therapy after I was diagnosed with multiple sclerosis I was increasing my intuition significantly. That is what is so mysterious about life. From a distance, it is sometimes difficult to discern what good can come from bad happenings and challenging events.

Chapter 31

Archetypal Energies: Releasing Spiritual Warrior, Shadow, Trickster, and Magician Archetypes for Healing

In this section, I want to show how thinking of yourself differently by developing a mythical name can help you tie into the exponentially power-enhancing effect of archetypal energies. These are latent thought patterns of energy you can mobilize to provide a lift into the higher levels of life and spirituality. These archetypes, or consciousness-connected patterns of thought, are described and explained thoroughly in my book, *Dreams: Guide to the Soul.*

After I was diagnosed with multiple sclerosis twenty-four years ago, I started in therapy with a Jungian dream analyst. This changed my life because I learned to tap into archetypal energies. The name given to me by a Native American in a dream was Life Force Dancer. I emblazoned this emblem on a T-shirt. The picture was of a Native American in what I thought of as dressed in traditional garb, dancing around a fire in a spiritual ceremony. This name was symbolic of the combination of energies that would help send my multiple sclerosis into remission.

I liked this image for several reasons. First, I thought of it as a spiritual warrior. There is a shadow archetype element that you must get in touch with to heal. The good side of the shadow wants to protect you (that is its primary job—self-defense) and will help you do whatever is necessary to heal.

You have to confront the illness and pledge to yourself to fight the good fight in spite of whatever may happen. You must be willing to use the warrior archetype, in the sense of being a spiritual warrior. I mean that in the most positive terms. You are fighting nature gone awry.

The image described above also involved the Magician archetype. The Native American is calling upon the Great Spirit. You are calling upon your own greater spirit or higher self to heal what you have been told cannot be healed. What you are trying to do will be magical if it occurs.

Native Americans were fond of the Trickster image. The essence of the Trickster is that he does things in an unconventional way. The Trickster archetype makes impossible situations work. Seeking conventional and unconventional means to heal, strengthened by the shadow to do whatever you have to, allows you to deal with an impossible disease like MS by making healing possible.

If you defeat multiple sclerosis, it is because you used the shadow in a positive way to promote healing. By tying into archetypal energies, you are increasing the force of your emotions, decisions, and actions by at least tenfold. You will win by summoning the energies of the Shadow, the spiritual Warrior, the Trickster, and the Magician. **YOU WILL HAVE FOUND HOW TO MIX CONFLICTING ENERGIES TOGETHER TO HEAL YOURSELF.** The world will benefit from your example of enduring persistent healing.

Chapter 32

Predictive Dreams

Dreams can be predictive. Clairvoyant or predictive dreams are one of the major categories or types of dreams. I give multiple examples of predictive dreams in my previous book, *Dreams: Guide to the Soul*. One of the most impressive predictive dreams I have personally known was created by my dreamer wife. It is seldom that a dream turns out to be this accurate in its predictions and connotations. I always knew my wife had something special going on with dreams. That is why I asked her to have a dream about how I should live so that I would heal. She had the dream, described in a previous chapter, of an angel appearing to her singing the four simple but transcendent rules for living that I was to follow to achieve healing.

She woke up one morning at about 5:30 and had that stunned look on her face whenever she has an amazing dream. I asked her if something was wrong. She said, "I just had a dream that seemed so real, it was like I was there." She described the dream as follows:

"I dreamed that Pete (the business manager at a private practice clinic where we both worked) was late for work. He came in at about 11 a.m. instead of his usual 8 a.m. because of a horrible accident. He came upon the aftermath of a severe accident several miles from the clinic. He was trying to help as much as he could. He pulled two dead bodies out of a car and helped the ambulance personnel. In the dream, I saw multiple crashes occurring all around the clinic later that same day."

I went to work and did not think too much about it; however, my memory of, and interest in, her dream increased once I arrived at work. Pete was missing. He finally came in around 11 a.m. I asked him why he was late. He replied, "I just pulled a dead pregnant woman out of a car." I thought to myself, those events fulfilled the two dead bodies predicted in my wife's dream. I thought we had better go out to lunch.

On the way to and from the restaurant from the clinic, we saw two car accidents. I had never seen a car accident when going to lunch with him previously. Later in the day, there was a loud collision of vehicles on the street right in front of the clinic. Because of that intense collision, a person died. Did I tell you that by now I was feeling spooked?

No one knows where predictions come from. Are some things fated? Do things become more fated as the past blends into the future and the antecedent events that lead to certain consequences set in stone? Is there a record of what will happen that gets written from the decisions we make in the here-and-now? My answers are maybe, yes, and yes. The decisions you and others make determine a large portion of the future. There are forces of nature that we can vaguely predict that adds a gambling probability of which events are likely to occur in a given person's life.

I think all the emotions, thoughts, actions, and decisions we make form what was thought of in ancient times as an Akashic record of fatalistic probability—we have created what interacts with nature, and the forces of the universe determine what is going to happen. What you do in the here-and-now really does determine the future. The probabilistic quantum theory that forces of nature make life a gamble means that all we can be sure of is what happens in the here-and-now.

Chapter 33

Meditation and Mantras

We met the great Yogi Bhajan in the early 1990s. He was about 64 back then. He had very strong opinions. He was also well educated, which I found out by winning a book at a random drawing at a supper for mental health professionals. There were various treatments offered for obsessive compulsive disorder (OCD) in the book. Each chapter showed a different treatment approach for OCD. Lo and behold, one of the chapters was by none other than Yogi Bhajan himself. What was interesting is that his approach was as successful as the other approaches. On second thought, it actually makes sense that his approach was successful—not surprising at all.

Obsessive compulsive disorder (OCD) results from an anxious person focusing on mostly irrelevant rituals and details so that she can forget about her underlying anxieties. The East, with its focus on mantras that are repeated over and over, would be a good model for refocusing the anxious obsessive energy on a compulsive ritual. The main difference is that the person is focusing on a higher purpose and spirituality rather than focusing on irrelevant detail such as colors of cars or the price of milk. Both methods work, only mantras seem to be spiritually healing and avoid excessively strange obsessive rituals, like making sure all your doors are locked, over and over. Mantras are obsessive about healing by doing a constructive, and, if you will, spiritual practice.

- The person repeating the mantra experiences some anxiety relief. She is doing something positive rather than trying to repetitively do some pointless behavior, such as repetitive hand-washing. The way the East uses the mantra can be viewed as a type of prayer or self-affirmation, which is a more constructive method of healing. I was instructed at a seminar by East-Indian physician Deepak Chopra to focus my meditation by silently thinking to myself "So-Hum." I think the reason for this sound was that it is inherently calming because it combines an element of "so what" combined with humming. It is almost impossible to be anxious while humming a happy tune. What you tell yourself matters psychologically, but the East takes this further.

The East knows that the mantra can have physical effects. For example, Meniere's disease is a constant ringing of the eardrums. By making the sound that "n" produces in a certain way (so that you feel the sound inside your head), the patient under his own will vibrates the eardrums. This sometimes can help a person learn to gain control over this irritating symptom.

Of course, the mantras are believed to have spiritual co-creative value. The great psychologist Wayne Dyer (who died in early September 2015) valued the manifestation aspect of mantras. He noticed that if you say the different religious names for God (Allah, Jehovah, Yahweh, and God), and if you hold the name and sound it out-loud, you will produce an "a" sound.

"A" just happens to be the first letter in the alphabet. Holding the "a" sound repeatedly for ten minutes or so by taking deep breaths and then letting out an "a" sound is invoking God to help you co-create what you are meditating upon. This particular out-loud sound mantra meditation is known as Japa in the East. It is different than other meditations. During meditation, it can sometimes be difficult to focus on one thing, and sometimes seem impossible to empty the mind. With Japa, you cannot empty your mind, but it is almost impossible not to focus on the one thing—breathing to make the "ahhhhhh" sound.

Eastern approaches and thinking feel good to me. The East generally regards the universe as God. The Dalai Lama was asked once what he thought regarding the creation of the universe. He responded that Buddhists mostly believe that what is here has always been here. He pointed out that if you posit a God, the question then becomes, who created God? At some point, in this view, one must accept that something has always been here. Buddhists nip it in the bud by assuming that what is here, has always been here. It makes stunning sense. A more parsimonious explanation like this is, to me, elegant logic.

I have been meditating the way Deepak Chopra recommended since I attended a two-day conference he gave in Phoenix. It was held at the Hyatt Hotel, which has a slowly rotating restaurant at the top of it. I have not found that it is beneficial to empty my mind. It is beneficial for me to focus on one thing. I think this focus helps me gain control of my attention and observe my mind from a distance. I suspect that if the person can get herself to do it, practicing focusing on one thing may help attention deficit—if the person can get herself to practice a meditation like this for twenty minutes or so per day.

The meditation recommended to the audience during the seminar was to spend about five minutes on each one of four words. The four words were *peace, harmony, laughter,* and *love.* When I am doing this, I take one word at a time, and repeat it over and over in my mind until I feel internally satisfied. The time length is not as important as the quality of focus is. Avoid checking the time. You want to focus on each one of these words, one by one, until you feel internally satisfied that the essence of the word has been ingrained in your subconscious. With practice, you will likely fall into a routine that solidifies the activity of focusing on the words in your mind the more you practice it. As you see the beneficial effect it has on your mood and behavior, in terms of being more relaxed, alert, and focused, your daily meditation sessions will be something to look forward to.

Chapter 34

The Roller Coaster of Emotional Transformation

Dealing with multiple sclerosis is working with major emotional transformation. As can be seen at the beginning of this book, my denial took the form of total repression. Once I was able to cognitively grasp the fact that I had multiple sclerosis, it was a matter of accepting the changes I needed to make in my life to get better. I think the total time of my repression was short, simply because it was presented to me with such hardcore evidence. There was no denying that I had multiple sclerosis. I had to figure out what I was going to do next to get better.

Early on, a lot of thoughts of "why me" occurred. In my mind, there were two ways of responding to this. One was based on spirituality. Maybe MS was part of God's plan for me. To take a more expanded view of spirituality, maybe it was what my spirit needed to experience in this life. There was some consolation in considering maybe this wasn't a completely random event. On the other hand, the notion that I had any participation in propelling this disaster upon my life was galling.

I did not know whether it was God's plan or my past soul's karma. Acceptance, for me, meant accepting that, regardless of how it came about, I indeed had it. But, after that acceptance, I had to do something about it. If you believe that this is a random universe, the question becomes irrelevant, because rather than asking "why me," you might as well be asking "why not me?"

It was hopeful that there were medications early on that were just being developed for multiple sclerosis. My multiple sclerosis started with hope. The positive results obtained from the new medications were hope delivered by the medical community. The promise of remission was delivered by an experimental combination of steroids with Cytoxan. Once these medications turned the tide, Tysabri and Ocrevus continued to improve my functioning by calling off the misguided immune system attacks and finding new neuronal pathways.

A lot of things from the early part of my life also helped me. My life is a story of hanging-in-there and doing-what-you-can under adverse circumstances. When there seems no reason to keep going, I learned early on in life how to put one foot in front of the other. The main message is to keep going, even if at that moment you can't see it going anywhere. For me, that is the definition of faith. The life experiences of harsh family circumstances, long-distance running, and extended educational endeavors taught me the value of hanging in there when the going gets tough. I believe patience and long-suffering will often save your life.

The first five years of having MS was for me a quiet and almost secretive period of my life. No one could really tell that I had multiple sclerosis who were not experienced MS observers. My balance was off, but not to the degree that people would notice. My speech was okay, and I could do entertainment with friends without anyone noticing. At that point, the way I described this vitality thief was that having MS felt more annoying than being nibbled to death by a duck. The duck will not succeed, but multiple sclerosis may take your life.

After having multiple sclerosis for six years, I entered the long-slow-slide phase. I began to feel like a frog in heated water that did not realize it was being cooked. My need to use a wheelchair in airports and the increasingly illegible scrawl of my writing was the "writing on the wall" of my deteriorated functioning. During this time, my wife and I went back to Cancun, Mexico, and Maui, Hawaii, to try to relive past glorious vacations. It, of course, did not work and only made the losses more painful.

I reached the point of becoming a true believer. But first I had to sink to the bottom and decide I didn't want to go down any further. I was ready to do anything positive and healing to keep from submerging any lower in that pit.

Early mornings became a sacred time for me. I was seeing Diana once a week and going to the physical therapy gym alone three times a week early in the morning. For me, there's something very quiet and special about early morning. The events of the day have not obscured my thinking yet. Long-term goals become clearer predawn. It was me, my thoughts, and my body working out that took the corrosive edge off worries.

Once I was to the point where I was noticing little improvements, I quietly steeled myself to pursue this disease. That was a major turning point that helped my enthusiasm and faith that the monster called MS could be defeated. I did not think there was one silver bullet that would bring multiple sclerosis down. I believed I needed a machine gun full of silver bullet treatments to stop MS before it sucked the life out of me.

Meditation and mindfulness kept me on course. I believe I had a sort of attention deficit caused by multiple sclerosis. My office manager thought I had "loseyitis." It was legend that you could hand something to Dr. Fox, and within two minutes it would be lost—and Dr. Fox will not have moved from the spot where you handed the item to him.

I found that to keep friendships and to avoid becoming isolated, I had to cut people a lot of slack as to how they talked to me about multiple sclerosis. People are simply curious. I realized I had to allow any questions from people about how MS affected me that were asked in good faith.

I got over feeling offended by realizing that people were not being offensive; they just did not know. Friends and most people ask questions to help them understand. The questions are a form of support. They would not ask if they did not care. If you do not give concerned people the chance to ask questions, they may start avoiding you. You hear less truth, because they may keep things from you to protect you. You begin to feel like a bomb. You do not want that. You may explode.

The computer served practical purposes, such as helping me find treatment methods, while also keeping my mind off the MS. It was something I could do well. It also helped me write my first book, which is probably something I'll be doing for the rest of my life. With MS, it is important to have choices for the future, because you never know where multiple sclerosis may take you. MS may be a passenger in your body vehicle through this journey in life, but don't allow MS to become your driver.

My emotions have become more labile, which is partially a biological effect, and partially the effect of the emotionally opening events occurring in your life because of MS. I realized even more sharply that I only have so much time in life. The things that enhance my life, I love more. On the other hand, I have no time for nonsense. As my current office manager puts it: "When Dr. Fox is mad, he's very mad. When he's happy, he's very happy."

It's amazing to see twenty-seven-year-old multiple sclerosis symptoms continue to turn around. Even today, I notice from time to time that an arm feels a little less numb or my writing improves a little bit more. People comment on my walking continuing to improve. I can even run if I must. Now, the only question is if I want to run. I'm in better health functionally than I was in my late 30s. Still, one must put aside the resentment for the years lost and the fun you could have had. Resentment must be replaced by a growing appreciation and joy over the common things I can do better than when I was younger.

I have stronger emotional reactions, especially to the people I am close to. Part of that is the MS, the other major part, or more major part, is that my wife died on July 31ˢᵗ of 2017. I am alone except for some friends and Debby's two cats. The cats and I always got along, but they were definitely Debby's cats. Now they act like I am the best thing. And it helps. At night, I have two cats that sleep on me. They never did that before. We now know we are survivors of a major, irreplaceable loss. It is funny how becoming closer to an animal makes one a better person.

My reaction to my wife's death was to plan a vacation to London, England. Christmas was always a special time for Debby. She had to encourage me to do the decorating and shopping. I now realize how much I liked and miss going shopping with her. Her favorite thing to do was to buy a gift for a cherished friend or relative. I had to do something to avoid Christmas. My ten days in London were interesting, and I met good people. I planned events for each day and saw many of the sights. I walked for miles each day. That was incomprehensible when I was fifty. I am now sixty-four. I feel like I am returning to my thirties' level of functioning.

Then there are just the events that I stop and marvel at almost every day. For instance, the reader probably would think nothing of carrying two glasses of water or a bowl of soup to a family room. Let me tell you, after I had multiple sclerosis for ten years, the idea of doing that was unthinkable. I know one of the major turning points was when I carried a dinner plate and a full glass of water for some distance. Debby leapt from her chair with tissues and anticipated the spillage.

After I glided into my chair, Debby could only say, "My God, you are getting better!"

I suppose my overwhelming happiness in that moment was not as great as an athlete's triumph after winning an Olympic gold medal, but it was close. Part of it is realizing that you are, indeed, returning to normal. For me, it felt like returning to being human. When fighting MS, I had an intense desire to return to the Self I had known most of my life.

Most of the MS years are faded memories that feel like watching a black-and-white movie in the distance at low volume. Too much repression can be negative. On the other hand, a certain amount of suppression is necessary to function in modern life.

If you allowed yourself no suppression and were fully cognizant at all times about what could happen, it would be very difficult to drive a car on a freeway, or perhaps even leave your home. That is what I found as a psychologist helping a client to get over PTSD from a car accident. I had to help him build up a resistance to the "what ifs." Catastrophic obsessing about what could happen is often the foundation upon which depression and anxiety build. Allow yourself mental vacations from the weight of multiple sclerosis.

It is no small point that I notice my balance and steadiness are much better. I have not had a major fall for at least ten years. I no longer have to carefully plan access to bathroom facilities like in the earlier MS days. Soiling my pants near a public setting is the closest I ever came to re-experiencing toddler shame for going potty where I was not supposed to.

My wife and I used to go on vacation to San Diego, California only, because it is a short, one-hour flight from Phoenix. It was the least stressful way for us to vacation. And avoiding stress is a huge part of successfully coping with multiple sclerosis. We both needed to be near a major medical center because of Debby's transplants and my MS. Our vacations were very restful and relaxing. It was a retreat to the beach and friends with some minor sightseeing. I have a desire to go to Europe more now that I can walk for miles. It was London in 2017; I have scheduled Rome for 2018; and I will probably go to Paris in 2019.

I realized how much I missed Debby when I was in London. My dreams were much more vivid and felt more real there. I think it is because seeing all the historic sights stimulates the dreamer's connection to the collective unconscious. The theory is that any thought any man has ever had is in the collective unconscious. This collective is like an internet of subconscious thought surrounding humanity. One of the signs that you are in deep connection with the collective unconscious is having dreams of classic historical sites.

One night I dreamed that we were together traveling. I reached over to what would have been her side of the bed, and, of course, she was not there. Tears are coming to my eyes as I write this because, as stupid as it sounds, I finally integrated cognitively, emotionally, and physically that she was dead and never to return. You can know things intellectually, but it takes time to integrate such a massive loss of love emotionally.

I have always been good at forming new relationships. I am not talking about seeking romantic involvement; I am talking about friendships. I cannot imagine molding myself completely to another person again. Once you know someone like that for years, you see the depths of who you are, especially if your mirror is a board-certified, empathic psychiatrist.

We seldom analyzed each other for fun; it was mostly in those moments when one was not seeing the whole picture. At those moments, you need someone you respect to tell you the truth. You must trust enough to discuss the most intimate feelings honestly and openly with someone who will kindly tell you what you need to hear, which is too often what you do not want to hear or refuse to see. Did I mention I was stubborn? It is the downside of being determined.

New relationships will have to be on a different basis. It will be more friendship and companionship than anything else. There is too much baggage to dump at someone's doorstep, although I may be willing to share a suitcase or two. It all depends on what the future brings, and I am living in the now.

For now, Debby became quite good friends with an ASU senior who was our office manager. She helped look after Debby in the final six months a lot. She still works as my office manager. Because of my wife's almost mother-daughter relationship with her, I am a sort of add-on pseudo-father figure. She has a biological father, who is great, thank you, so the fatherly feelings are all on my part. To her, I am a tolerable boss who has good and less-than-good days.

My dilemma of not having traveling companions has been partially solved. She, her sixteen-year-old brother, and I plan to travel to Rome. If it works out, we may take more journeys. It is massive sightseeing, and it is funky. I have always liked funky. These days, I am all about taking one step at a time and not looking too far into the future. As I get older, I am more hesitant to buy green bananas. The time horizon of predicting future events has become shorter as I come closer to the inevitable event horizon of death.

I mainly hope what happens after death coincides with my spirituality and is not a black hole sucking the life out of the universe. On the other hand, if there were nothing after death, would it make any difference? I mean, I do not remember any previous lives, and I am not particularly fascinated with the concept. A psychic told me once that I may have been a lieutenant for the North in the Civil War. The story she told was that on a particular battle, I became aware that my men had raped, burned, and pillaged. Instead of doing something about it, I simply ordered the men to charge on to the next battle in hot pursuit of the retreating Confederates. I guess it could explain the beatings I received in this life.

If that is the case, it makes me wonder what karmic consequences I may have to endure in the next life theoretically. The upside of reincarnation is that you keep coming back for another life until you get it right and achieve nirvana. I can feel glimpses of it rarely when I meditate.

This life seems too short and sometimes too long in a great paradoxical double bind. I like the ideas of continual learning and being given a zillion chances to get it right, which is the heart of reincarnation. It does bring up interesting questions such as *What does karma do with Adolf Hitler?* I guess a fitting scenario might involve coming back as an insect six million times. Of course, how does one behave as a good insect?

The question occurs to all people who are diagnosed with multiple sclerosis, namely, Why me? Thinking that somehow it was planned for your own good is a hard pill to swallow. I thought I would never say this because I hated MS so much, but for me there has been a lot of good to come from it.

I think the solution to most MS challenges follows a different course for each person. We are all different with different histories and different ways of handling stress. There will be some commonalities, but you have to find the particular, and the many things that may work for you at this particular time in your life. You may wish to adopt a rule such as trying anything that has a 10% chance of working. You will need to adjust that risk percentage higher or lower according to your situation and risk tolerance. For me, it meant trying almost anything that did not involve a high risk of permanent damage. Based on this rule, I did not feel that I was risking anything but temporary discomfort. Fortunately, in my case, enduring multiple transient discomforts helped me get rid of a seemingly permanent disability.

There continue to be reminders of the battles I fought and the war with multiple sclerosis that was won. I still have a sticker in my car that allows me to park in handicapped parking if need be.

After all, multiple sclerosis is a permanent disability with an inevitable downhill course, right? Sometimes I have to smile thankfully; other times I am giddy. It all depends on how MS is affecting me that day. Is multiple sclerosis an unmitigated disaster? I can firmly state, "It depends."

It depends on you—whether you can fight it; whether you want to fight it; and whether you are to the point that you have taken all reasonable measures for you. But even then, I would urge you to keep your eyes on MS research and treatment. We are living in the Star Trek age of medicine where the great monsters of illness are starting to be tamed. In the words of Dylan Thomas, whose father was, at the time Dylan wrote this, reportedly going blind and dying:

Do not go gentle into that good night.

Rage, rage against the dying of the light.

Chapter 35

My MS Diet, Vitamins, and Favorite Drugs

The diet aspect is relatively simple. It mostly involves avoiding foods that stimulate your immune system. For me, this means mostly a gluten-free diet. Being raised on a farm, I know that wheat is subject to more molds, fungi, and diseases than other grains. I believe some of this goes into the wheat we eat. I believe it stimulates the immune system, and the immune system of the person with MS overreacts to the wheat molds and ends up errantly attacking the person's nervous system as well. However, this is only one of several examples of why wheat is not good for us. Many problems involve the different ways of farming and the wheat seed that is used.

There is another issue with wheat, from what I have been told. The reader is forewarned that my conclusions have not been scientifically verified as having been shown to have negative effects on consumers. I have been told and have read that nowadays the big corporate farmers douse the wheat with chemicals (Roundup), which increases production, because the wheat strives to make more seed right before it dies. They also spray the wheat with Roundup once the seeds have formed so that the wheat can be harvested.

If you have thousands of acres of wheat, you need to get it harvested as quickly as you can—it sometimes rains so much that the wheat cannot be harvested. By using Roundup, the number of bushels of wheat produced per acre increases, and you do not have to worry about being rained out and unable to harvest the wheat in a timely fashion. Unfortunately, Roundup is quite toxic. In many ways, Roundup can be thought of as watered-down Agent Orange. I think if you eat a lot of wheat, you may be giving yourself a micro-dose of a toxic chemical. Wheat has been made unhealthy. I have been told the above by a large corporate farmer, plus there is information on the internet and in books and recent studies, such as what follows.

As the Healthy Home Economist succinctly summarized at her informative website, http://www.thehealthyhomeeconomist.com/real-reason-for-toxic-wheat-its-not-gluten/:

> A common wheat harvest protocol in the United States is to drench the wheat fields with Roundup several days before the combine harvesters work through the fields as the practice allows for an earlier, easier and bigger harvest.

There is also the idea that genetically modified wheat is fooling around with a food—wheat—that has been around for millennia, on a fundamental level. The wheat today is different from what it was one hundred years ago. These differences may have a significant impact on how effectively humans are able to digest wheat, and the effects it may have on our biological organism as a whole, including our immune system.

The primary culprit is wheat, but other grains, such as barley and rye, can also have this effect on me (to a somewhat lesser degree in my case). Corn and rice are safe for me as I have never had a reaction to these grains (and notice that they do not contain gluten, which may also be part of the reason they do not affect me).

I avoid the obvious wheat products such as bread, pasta, pastries, and pretty much all bakery goods. Fortunately, one can almost always find substitutes that use corn, rice, or some other non-gluten grain like quinoa or vegetables like potatoes or peas. Many grocery stores carry gluten-free products, and many have gluten-free sections in their stores. An ever-increasing number of restaurants are now offering gluten-free dishes and/or guidance as to which dishes are gluten-free.

When shopping, one must carefully scan the ingredients contained in each food to make sure it does not contain wheat or wheat flour. I am a vegetarian to some degree, but I feel like I need heavy-duty protein from time to time. I will occasionally eat red meat, but only occasionally. You can get considerable protein from nuts, beans, and legumes. I also eat fish and invariably try to eat wild salmon in restaurants whenever I can.

Again, with my farm background, I am aware of the various medicines and cattle additives that enter the meat supply, which may stimulate an already overly reactive immune system that a person with multiple sclerosis has. Chicken is probably less prone to harboring medicines, mainly because their life span is so short that there is less time for the offending medicines to build up in their meat and fat. Fat is where most toxic materials are stored.

Cattle meat has significantly more fat than chicken, which is why it probably has more of an effect on the immune system. We do need some fat in our diet, as a thin layer of fat covers our immune system. My favorite source of fat is salmon because the fat we gain from salmon is High Density Lipid (HDL) fat—the good fat.

If we do not have enough HDL fat in our system, our body will make nervous system parts out of Low Density Lipid (LDL) fat—the bad fat. Therefore, we want to give up or only occasionally eat fast food. These foods are often full of LDL greasy fat. We call fast food junk food because that is literally what we are making body parts out of when we eat fast food—junk. I do not want my body parts and nervous system to be constructed from McDonald's, Burger King, etc. Have it your way and give yourself a break from the weak fats these establishments proffer.

Candy should be eaten in moderation—when you eat too much, it makes you hyper. Sugar increases inflammation, and you do not want inflammation because that is a hallmark of MS. As you can tell, I take it easy on sugar because I think in moderation it helps my activity level, and fatigue is a big part of MS. Also, there is no denying that sugar is a major contributor to food tasting good.

Caffeine in excess will also make you hyper unless you have attention deficit, in which case it has no effect, or the opposite, sedating, effect. I think it could be possible that foods like this in excess, if they make you hyper, also will make the MS person's immune system hyperactive. This is not a good thing as the immune system may use its hyperactivity to set off a round of mistakenly attacking your nervous system in its haste to over-defend you. More important than any of the above, caffeine stimulates anxiety. You do not want to use caffeine if you have high levels of anxiety or panic attacks.

Eating fruits and vegetables cannot be emphasized enough. This is the surest and best way to get essential vitamins, minerals, and body-building substances unique to plants and some animals that we do not totally understand. The chances of getting Alzheimer's was reduced by a dramatic 76% in a study at Vanderbilt University by people drinking a glass of any vegetable or fruit juice three times per week (Carper 2010).

Taking vitamins is necessary, especially when you have MS, to avoid deficiencies that can make the consequences of the illness worse. Vitamins B and D are especially important. Vitamin B is important because it is vital to the nervous system. Vitamin D is important—in fact, it's possible that vitamin D may be protective or delay the onset of multiple sclerosis.

One way to get your body to produce massive amounts of vitamin D is to expose your body to the sun. Your body can typically make massive amounts of vitamin D from exposure to sunlight. People in northern latitudes and cold climates get MS significantly more often. This is probably partially due to being exposed to less sun. Immune systems in northern latitudes are also probably more likely to change from more frequent exposure to pathogens (viruses, bacteria, colds, etc.).

Regarding vitamin B, it is important for people with MS to take medication that carries vitamin B across the blood-brain barrier. You need a prescription to get medication that does that. Cerefolin NAC (the generic is metafolbic plus RF) is a doctor-prescribed medication or medical food that delivers vitamin B to the brain, which is the most important place in need of repair because of the neuronal demyelinating effects of multiple sclerosis. It is a pill that you take once per day. I believe Cerefolin NAC helps preserve cognitive functioning.

Until recently, there was no medication to directly reverse peripheral neuropathy. With MS, the demyelinating of neurons in the body leads to the peripheral neuropathy symptoms of numbness and difficulty moving. I have greatly improved my ability to move (MS is considered a movement disorder).

Numbness in my extremities has been reduced from 40% to 60% down to 5% to 20%. The reason for the variation in the estimates is because MS changes from day to day depending upon how well the body is either repairing or not repairing neural damage. The saying with MS is that if you do not like the symptoms, hold on. This saying is true because MS symptoms are virtually always likely to change.

The numbness is an annoying, but manageable, symptom. The main thing the numbness affected for me was the legibility of my writing. How well I write is a significant marker of how I am doing. My writing has continued to improve steadily, which I think is due to my medication, mind, physical therapy, diet, and Eastern practices.

I take Metanx (the generic is Foltanx), which is a very high-dose vitamin B that has been shown to reduce peripheral neuropathy. You also need a doctor's prescription to get this medication or medical food because it crosses the blood-brain barrier. Metanx is taken twice a day typically.

I also want to mention Wellbutrin (the generic is Bupropion). It is an antidepressant with almost all positive side effects. When it was being tested on around 5,000 patients, 40% of people taking

Wellbutrin stopped smoking without anyone saying anything about stopping smoking to them. Now, 60% did not stop smoking, but a substantial minority did without any intervention. Smokers I have talked to that it worked on tell me that it changed the taste of the cigarette so that they were no longer interested. When it is used to stop smoking, it is labeled as Zyban. A warning on the bottle says not to use Zyban with Wellbutrin. That is because Zyban is Wellbutrin.

The effect of Wellbutrin is to increase the body's neurotransmitter, dopamine. You use dopamine whenever you think or use a muscle. It improves attention to the point that it can be used for adult attention deficit. It makes a person more alert and focused while reducing depression.

Wellbutrin also usually improves sex because it increases dopamine levels. You use dopamine to move muscles. Most people move a muscle or three when having sex.

The only side effect I have heard about is that it can reduce seizure threshold. For that reason, people prone to having seizures would not want to take Wellbutrin. Alcohol and illegal drugs that reduce seizure threshold should not be used when taking Wellbutrin.

Other than that, which of the many antidepressants is likely to work with a given person should be assessed and evaluated by your medical doctor. Multiple sclerosis is a stress that makes it more likely that a person will become depressed. The antidepressant that reduces depression the most and has the least side effects for a person is the right antidepressant for that person. You want to do more than go natural when fighting the demonic thief of life known as multiple sclerosis. There is nothing natural about your immune system deciding to attack your body. That process is anti-nature and anti-life. Consider everything at your disposal to stop that attack.

Chapter 36

Teeth

The main idea behind most of the different avenues I pursued to try to send the multiple sclerosis into remission involved doing whatever I could to keep from activating my immune system. There are two major ways my immune system has been activated during the fifteen years the MS was active. One was when I had periodontal disease which became worse when I developed MS. The other is when I get a cold.

I developed periodontal disease in my mid-thirties. I was told that there was not very much that could be done about it. It reminds me of MS because I was told that there was not much you could do about MS. I guess it assures some people that there is nothing they can try doing to get better. I take no consolation from being told there is nothing I can do. My response to that dreary news goes something like, "Oh, yeah?!!"

I started looking at the ingredients in toothpaste and noticed that many appeared to have peroxide-like components. I subsequently stumbled upon a study by a doctor in Africa who indicated that when he ran low on supplies, he used hydrogen peroxide as a disinfectant. I reasoned that periodontal disease was an infection and that disinfectant should help combat it.

I mixed hydrogen peroxide with water so that half was water and half was hydrogen peroxide. Do not drink the hydrogen peroxide under any circumstances! You may want to dilute the hydrogen peroxide more than I do because I suspect I have a high tolerance for hydrogen peroxide—perhaps dilute it to two or three parts water to one part hydrogen peroxide. I brush my teeth twice per day. (I think brushing your teeth more than that is excessive and can actually do some harm to the enamel, especially if you brush hard.) I assume that you are using an electric toothbrush since it does such a better job than a non-electric toothbrush.

After each brushing, I swished the solution around my mouth for about a minute after each brushing. After a month, my teeth were a shade whiter. After six months, my teeth were five shades brighter. After a year, I no longer had periodontal disease. My dentist was surprised.

Gradually, as problems developed with my teeth, I had all the mercury amalgam fillings removed and replaced with white material. It may have been a coincidence, but removal of my last deep mercury filling coincided with when my MS symptoms started to dramatically improve. I'm just saying . . .

Multiple sclerosis is an autoimmune disease that is inflammatory, like other autoimmune diseases such as Alzheimer's, rheumatism, Parkinson's, rheumatoid arthritis, lupus, eczema, diabetes, etc. It made sense to me that as I got rid of the periodontal disease inflammation, it might help reduce my MS inflammation. At the very least, the inflammation that was caused by periodontal disease would no longer aggravate the multiple sclerosis.

You want to get rid of inflammations in your body to fight MS. Multiple sclerosis can be expected to react like other inflammatory autoimmune diseases such as Alzheimer's. UCLA found that people who had periodontal teeth disease before age 35, quadrupled the risk of dementia when they were elderly (Carper 2010).

You want to avoid other diseases that can stimulate your immune system such as colds and flu. For this reason, it is important to be vaccinated to avoid getting sick. Having colds or flu repeatedly may be one of the causes of MS if having repeated illnesses like this modifies the immune system. Although there may be drawbacks to some vaccinations, the main thing is to make sure you use vaccines that do not have the live form of the virus. Most vaccines use dead virus, but some do use live virus (such as FluMist). In my mind, you want to avoid live virus for two reasons:

1. You do not want to overstimulate the immune system.

2. Most people with MS need to take medication (such as Avonex, Betaseron, Copaxone, Tysabri, Tecfidera, Ocrevus, etc.) that reduces the ability of the immune system to fight viruses. You do not want to fight a live virus with a reduced immune system. It is advisable not to have contact with people who have been vaccinated with a live virus (such as FluMist) for about a month.

Handshaking is a major transmitter of disease. One study found that you were more likely to acquire a disease from handshaking than if you hugged the other person. That is because the hands are most likely to touch entry points to the human body where disease can fester. I think the Japanese custom of slightly bowing to each other makes more sense. I wonder if that social custom came into popularity because the Japanese witnessed plagues ravage their civilization and were smart enough to consider that handshaking was a contributor to spreading diseases.

Handshaking is an old, established social practice that seems impossible to stop. Sometimes even I cannot avoid shaking hands when I know the person involved would not understand why I am not shaking his hand or would take it as an insult. I am committed to simply say, "I do not shake hands" without giving excuses, and it is getting easier to do so.

Chapter 37

My Exercise Habits

Throughout high school, I did chores on the dairy farm twice a day, for a total of four hours per day. I also worked eight to fourteen hours per day on weekends depending upon the season. To try to maintain myself and have a life outside of "the farm," I insisted on being a long-distance runner. I know the above sounds like "When I was young, I walked ten miles through five feet of snow to get to school," but it is the truth.

Cross country and track were my vacation from school and the farm. I typically ran approximately five to eight miles per day in-season, and two to five off-season. My usual event in these sports was about two miles long. During college, I continued my off-season practice and understood well the runner's high. During long-distance runs, endorphins often flood your body, which literally can make you high. These natural pain killers are a response to the damage the runner is inflicting on his muscles.

I now think that stair-stepping at the gym is preferable to running in many ways. In long-distance running, you are throwing your body into the air, and then crashing down on your legs, knees, feet, and toes. I once pulled a knee ligament that largely sidelined me for six months. I had constant sores on my feet and toes that I had to guard from infection. I decided some time ago to reduce running past the age of fifty. In any case, long-distance running has blessed me with seemingly permanent low blood pressure.

My routine now is to lift weights one to three times per week alongside at least ten minutes on a stair-stepping machine. I need to do yoga once or twice per week. I follow daily exercises that my cranial-sacral physical therapist assigns to me. These exercises usually prevent back pain. They also work on coordinating the left side of my body with the right side. The multiple sclerosis mainly attacked my right side, and there are imbalances that need to be better coordinated. Also, I started walking more, mostly at the insistence of Debby, whose endurance at walking down an ocean beach was remarkable considering all her health challenges. I am integrating short daily walks into my life, as walking seems to help everything and hurts nothing.

Chapter 38

My Prayer Routine

Readers may be interested in my actual prayer routine. This routine is based on how I was raised, with a certain religious and spiritual template. It is easier to turbocharge knowledge with which I was raised, with additions based on my experience, than it would be to create a whole new system. My imagination has not been field-tested on millennia of human experience like ancient religions have.

I will describe the structure of my prayer routine so that people can adapt and change it according to their religious views and needs. I urge you to develop your own angels, icons, and saints according to your beliefs. The structure of my prayer routine is as follows:

1. First, I pray for the help of the Big Three archangels, **Archangel Michael, Archangel Rafael,** and **Archangel Gabriel.**

2. Next, I include the celestial and major angels, which, in my case, are **Azrael,** the angel of death; **Jophiel,** the angel of beauty; **Metatron,** who in my mind is the writer's angel; **Raziel,** the angel of divine wisdom; **Ariel,** the angel of nature; and last, but certainly not least, **Jeremiel,** the angel who provides assistance in understanding dreams.

3. Next, I pray for help in appealing to God to what I call everyday angels (guardian angel, personal healing angel, helper angel, teacher angel, joy angel, master guide, and runner angel).

4. I then pray for intercession assistance from saints and icons (Saint Teresa, Saint Francis, Saint Germaine, Padre Pio, Jesus Christ, and Buddha).

5. Next I pray for help from deceased relatives, friends, and long-term patients who died due to disease. I also include personal doctors, teachers, and professors who had a significant positive effect on me.

6. I then list the things that I want to manifest in my life. Healing for myself and people close to me is paramount, but I do also list any concerns I have regarding life decisions.

7. I finish the invocation for miracles in my life by repeating what Saint Teresa said in her prayers: "Please ask God to grant me the gifts I implore, and tell God that I will love him/her each day more and more."

8. I then repeat a saying from Shakti Gawain in her book *Creative Visualization*: "This or something better now manifests for me in completely positive and harmonious ways, for the highest good of all involved."

9. I then say some standard prayers that were taught to me when I was young (the Our Father, Hail Mary, and Glory Be—this threesome repeated five times).

This is very personal; prayer is born from personal spirituality. The above is my unique prayer routine, which may not apply to you. You must develop your own routine according to your beliefs, so that you harness the full power of your subconscious. The reader is encouraged to include and/or substitute whatever prayers you usually say in respect to your beliefs.

Chapter 39

The Important Things

As a psychologist, having known thousands of people at a deep level, I believe the most important thing is one's attitude about life and fate. Are certain things fated? Do we have a certain amount of free will? For me, the answer is yes. Let me explain.

I believe, and science has shown, the universe is constructed on a probabilistic basis. Whatever you think or do goes into a quantum mix that feeds into the collective unconscious. The whole of quantum physics provides strong support for outcomes to be only a probability determined by the surrounding conditions. I believe a major part of those conditions is the attitudes and personality of the person. I think this is especially true in the case of physical health.

The mind is in direct contact with your health always. It is not the gas that powers the body; it is more like the oil. When it gets dirty, it needs to be changed. New and strong healthy attitudes are like clean oil—the body will then run a lot smoother. You will need to do physical exercise such as yoga or working out or an enjoyable physical activity to keep you grounded and in contact with how you are physically functioning.

One thing virtually every person with multiple sclerosis will be told is that he needs to accept MS. To me, it depends on whether you view acceptance as an excuse to sit back, declare disability, and passively go into the dark night of decline ending with death, or whether you decide to fight it. While you fight it, it is acceptance to realize that healing is against all odds. Faith is the decision to do whatever you can to improve the odds, no matter how dire the situation. It is the stuff out of which miracles are made.

The part of you that fights for health needs to be in close contact with your own shadow. The shadow is the aggressive part of you that fights for health. It, of course, needs to be guided by the other parts of your personality so that no harm is done to others or to yourself.

You need the shadow to be assertive with others about what you need to get better. You need to be assertive with yourself to take the necessary health-promoting steps. Your shadow is what gives you resolve of steel. Your determination to be patient and long-suffering despite the odds against you is what will carry the day.

How long should you carry on the fight? In my view, as long as humanly possible for you. This will be different for each person depending on individual character and circumstances.

There is a time to "give up the fight," which is when death is imminent, and continued suffering becomes unbearable. My wife and I had living wills. When the point of no return has been reached, and the comatose person can live only with the help of machines—that is the point to allow the loved one to die and stop the pain, in my view.

I am not saying that we want to ignore fate in hopeless cases. In my case, having a 5% chance of recovering was good enough odds to continue the fight. I fortunately had the emotional support, material support, and inner resolve to carry on the struggle. You must develop the character to persevere, and in turn, engage in the quest for health, which will strengthen your determination. Having at least one or several people who are vitally committed to your survival because they love you is invaluable. Social support will often help your willpower to exert the effort to do things you would not otherwise do, such as exercise.

I had a certain amount of engrained stubbornness, which I put to good use. Early on, when I was often receiving the message that I should passively accept the MS, I could not help but think, "I hope I am never completely comfortable with the symptoms." If there was a fighting chance, I was willing to believe that fighting multiple sclerosis could be successful. That is another main thing—you must be willing to fight against the odds. It helps if you cultivate standing up for what you believe.

Reflecting on these matters had the surprising effect of realizing how much my spirituality improved the likelihood that I could recover much of my prior Self. My survival, in the end, turned out to be a soul issue. I learned that I am the best assessor of what is likely to work for me. Getting in touch with my intuition through meditation, dream interpretation, and psychotherapy was vital in helping me choose what course of treatments I should follow. Listen to your inner voice. In a person of reasonable mental health and intelligence, it is virtually never wrong.

Having "come out the other end," in my journey to heal from multiple sclerosis, it is vital to forgive people who have mistreated you. Carrying grudges about the past simply depletes your energy and will do you no good. I am not forgiving them because it was all right what they did, or because I approve of them as people. I forgive them because they are not worth my precious energy anymore. Carrying grudges requires energy. I am simply reclaiming the energy stolen from me and refusing to give them anymore.

Lastly, you need reasons to live. My main desire was to live a good life, to have people I love and people who love me. I simply want to be a good person. When I have regrets about my life, it usually amounts to wishing I had been a better person or treated people better. I think I do not have too many regrets, but there are always ways we can improve ourselves and, consequently, the world.

Being a psychologist, I have always believed that thought was, as Albert Einstein said, the most powerful force in the universe. Healing from multiple sclerosis is due to the mind and spirit bending against an intruder that we no longer want as part of our life. This recuperation makes the dramatic point that we must realize that we oversee our body and soul. The spirit I am trying to convey is best expressed in the following poem by William Ernest Henley (1849–1903):

Invictus: The Unconquerable

Out of the night that covers me,

Black as the pit from pole to pole,

I thank whatever gods may be

For my unconquerable soul.

In the fell clutch of circumstance

I have not winced nor cried aloud.

Under the bludgeonings of chance

My head is bloody, but unbowed.

Beyond this place of wrath and tears

Looms but the Horror of the shade,

And yet the menace of the years

Finds, and shall find me, unafraid.

It matters not how strait the gate,

How charged with punishments the scroll,

I am the master of my fate:

I am the captain of my soul.

The poem is a monument to carrying on for a purpose that is positive and just. It was what I had to believe to persevere. Only you can decide if this course is right for you.

The major change that has occurred in my life is that I have a profound feeling of gratefulness for common things like being able to walk through a crowd without falling because of the slight and quick shifts in weight that must be made to each leg as we maneuver our way through the crowd. MS brings into sharp relief the fact that anything can be taken from us at any time in this life. It makes me want to go out and explore the world more in terms of traveling.

The self-reliance and independent functioning that I prefer when traveling would have been unimaginable in my MS days. Words cannot adequately express how I notice that I talk about my MS days as if it were ancient history. I must remember that I still technically have multiple sclerosis. Warding off this disease is still a major part of my life, but now it is a life I can live with!

Chapter 40

Transcendent Experiences

For me, 2017 will always be the year of intense and almost otherworldly experiences. After Debby's death, her sister asked me if I had had any unusual or spiritual-like experiences. I thought about it and said that Debby told me to have compassion for others. That was it. That was the main thing—show compassion to others. I experienced this as if she was looking at me and talking to me. I stopped and thought about it and realized that this was more of a vision than anything. She was on life support and had tubes down her throat and there is no way she could have talked to me, let alone even looked my way.

We had such a deep spiritual connection, that I just accepted that this was happening and considered it as nothing unusual. I now realize I was either in a state of shock, or I had had a spiritual vision. In my world, I now favor the latter explanation. I think her family would verify that I was of sound mind at the time, although I was stressed, of course.

We sometimes did the tarot cards at home for entertainment. It was always interesting to see what they would say. There may be something going on with the tarot cards, and even if there isn't, it can still be valuable to do them because I believe you get more in touch with your subconscious about how you feel towards the particular question. It's sort of a self-Rorschach, if you will. The Rorschach is a projective personality test that makes inferences about a person's perceptions of what she sees in a set of inkblots. When I'm "interpreting" the tarot cards, it feels a little bit like projective interpretation, but, of course, the Rorschach is based on a much more reliable and proven set of previously gathered extensive research.

I seem to have a connection now to Debby through the cards. I seldom do the cards, but if I do, I sometimes can visualize Debby's response to the question as either a smile, or by looking down, shrugging her shoulders, or shaking her head. Debby was not shy about expressing her opinion.

The second unusual occurrence was my first direct experience of time slowing down during a traumatic event. I was driving my car about forty miles per hour, when a car on the side street pulled out directly in front of me, about fifteen feet in front of me. I didn't have time for my foot to even reach the brake pedal.

The collision occurred in the blink of an eye. It felt like it occurred over the course of at least a minute, maybe two minutes. I remember realizing that I was in an accident, and then seeing the other car, which was a large SUV, roll over in front of me. The other vehicle landed on its roof. What is even more remarkable is that neither one of us was hurt. Both vehicles were totaled. The other driver was cited for a failure to yield.

The airbag exploding in front of me seemed like a breath of fresh air. I actually wondered if I had died because everywhere I looked was covered by white from the airbag. I was brought to reality by a cop kicking open the passenger door after I unlocked it.

My life has been spared at least three separate times by technology and medical wonders. I had my appendix out just before it was ready to explode when I was twenty-eight. Modern medicine was largely responsible for turning around the MS. Automotive technology saved my life, and the other driver's life. I am very fortunate to be living in the 21st century. The thing is, I wouldn't want to live in the past, and the future is dicey because of wars between nations which have to stop. I am very happy to have lived in the time that I have. Overall, life has been good to me.

Epilogue

Much has happened in the time since I wrote many of the previous chapters. My beloved wife of thirty-two years, Debby Brogan, died at the age of sixty-one on July 31st of 2017. It was predicted, before we were married, that she probably would not make it to the age of forty. Her love of life, tenacity, and wisdom will not be forgotten by many people. She was an awe-inspiring woman and doctor who schooled me in how to take care of myself properly.

Also, there has been a major change of medication in the treatment of my multiple sclerosis, which I'm very happy about. Tysabri was changed to Ocrevus. Tysabri was an infusion that I took every six to eight weeks. Ocrevus is an infusion that lasts for six months. Only two infusions are necessary per year. Yay!

Multiple sclerosis is like a fifty-pound weight that you have to balance on your head constantly. To have to think about MS less is like a gift from God. Having to dwell on multiple sclerosis too much saps your energy.

The problem with Tysabri is it can allow the JC virus to be activated, which can potentially cause lesions on the brain. I was always JC-negative during the ten years or so that I took it, so there was no danger. At the end of 2017, I had a test that was JC-positive. I was told that it was possible to turn it negative again, which is what happened. The next blood test was JC-negative.

Nevertheless, I was told about Ocrevus, which appears not to have the potential dangerous side effect of the JC virus. From the research I've read, it seems to have less adverse effects on the immune system. In any case, the research on Ocrevus is overall better.

In fact, it is the only medication approved for primary progressive multiple sclerosis, which is the type I have. So, I will once again have the new and current 800-pound-gorilla-MS-medication. I had my first

Ocrevus infusion in December of 2017. After twenty-seven years of MS, a new chapter of treatment begins. Charge!

Since the 1990s, a corner was turned in multiple sclerosis research that is reaching a better understanding of the disease. It is likely that the MS sufferer will likely see many positive and life-changing treatments in their lifetime as I have. I am so grateful, words cannot express it.

References

Byrd, R.C. (1988). Positive therapeutic effects of intercessory prayer in a coronary care unit population. **Southern Medical Journal, 81,** 826–9.

Carper, J. (2012). 100 Simple Things You Can Do to Prevent Alzheimer's and Age-Related Memory Loss. New York, NY: Little, Brown and Company.

Choudhury, B. & Goldstein, J. (2000). **Bikram's Beginning Yoga Class.** New York, NY: J. P. Tarcher.

Dossey, L. (1995). Healing Words: The Power of Prayer and the Practice of Medicine. New York, NY: Harper One.

Dossey, L. (2014). One Mind: How Our Individual Mind Is Part of a Greater Consciousness and Why It Matters. Carlsbad, CA: Hay House.

Fox, S.G. (2013). **Dreams: Guide to the Soul.** Mesa, AZ: Steven G. Fox. Printed by CreateSpace.

Fox, S.G., & Walters. H.A. (1986). The impact of general versus specific expert testimony and eyewitness confidence upon mock juror judgment. **Law and Human Behavior, 10,** 215-228.

Gawain, S. (2002). Creative Visualization: Use the Power of Your Imagination to Create What You Want in Your Life. Nataraj: New World Library.

Henley, W. E. (1900). Invictus: The Unconquerable. **Poems** (Fourth ed.). London: David Nutt. 119.

Lipton, B. H. (2008). The Biology of Belief: Unleashing the Power of Consciousness, Matter, & Miracles. Carlsbad, CA: Hay House.

Meier, M.H., Caspi, A., Amber, A., et al. (2012). Persistent cannabis users show neuropsychological decline from childhood to midlife. **Proceedings of the National Academy of Sciences.** Epub E2657-64.

Schucman, H. (1992). **A Course in Miracles.** Mill Valley, CA: Foundation for Inner Peace.

Thomas, D. (1979). Do Not Go Gentle Into That Good Night. Shawnee Press.

Tolle, E. (2004). **The Power of Now: A Guide to Spiritual Enlightenment.** Vancouver, Canada: Namaste Publishing.

Woodman, M. (1989). **The Ravaged Bridegroom.** Toronto, Canada: Inner City Books.

Acknowledgements

I am alive because of my beloved and deceased wife, Debby. I want to thank my special sisters, Lolly and Valois, for helping me preserve my mental health. I want to forgive my brothers for their abuse, as I am doing well. In the end, they only hurt themselves.